A THERAPIST'S GUIDE TO
ART THERAPY ASSESSMENTS

ABOUT THE AUTHOR

Stephanie L. Brooke is a private practitioner in Rochester, New York. She received training as an art therapist at Hillside Children's Center in Geneseo, New York. Ms. Brooke conducts individual, couples, and group counseling for women's interests. Specifically, she specializes in sexual abuse issues. Additionally, Ms. Brooke is a psychology and human relations instructor at Geneseo Community College in Lakeville, New York. For the past 15 years, she has been dedicated pastel painter.

A THERAPIST'S GUIDE TO ART THERAPY ASSESSMENTS
Tools of the Trade

By

STEPHANIE L. BROOKE, M.S., N.C.C.

With a Foreword by

Harriet Wadeson, Ph.D., A.T.R.

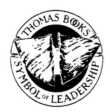

CHARLES C THOMAS • PUBLISHER, LTD.
Springfield • Illinois • U.S.A.

Published and Distributed Throughout the World by

CHARLES C THOMAS • PUBLISHER • LTD
2600 South First Street
Springfield, Illinois 62794-9265

© *1996 by* CHARLES C THOMAS • PUBLISHER • LTD
ISBN 0-398-06618-3 (cloth)
ISBN 0-398-06619-1 (paper)
Library of Congress Catalog Card Number: 96-11642

With THOMAS BOOKS *careful attention is given to all details of manufacturing
and design. It is the Publisher's desire to present books that are satisfactory as to their
physical qualities and artistic possibilities and appropriate for their particular use.*
THOMAS BOOKS *will be true to those laws of quality that assure a good name
and good will.*

Printed in the United States of America
SC-R-3

Library of Congress Cataloging-in-Publication Data

Brooke, Stephanie L.
    A therapist's guide to art therapy assessments : tools of the
trade / by Stephanie L. Brooks ; with a foreword by Harriet Wadeson.
        p.   cm.
    Includes bibliographical references and index.
    ISBN 0-398-06618-3 (cloth).—ISBN 0-398-06619-1 (paper)
    1. Art therapy.   2. Projective techniques.   I. Title.
RC489.A7B75   1996
616.89'1656—dc20
                                                              96-11642
                                                                  CIP

FOREWORD

Among the most controversial and misunderstood aspects of art therapy are interpretations of the art and its corollary, assessment. Art expression can be so seductive and the investigator's wish "to know" so strong that one can readily project meaning into the art of another. Clinician colleagues, perhaps a bit mystified and awed by the world of art, may look to the art therapist as possessor of the rosetta stone to decode the hieroglyphics of clients' images. Such can be heady expectations an art therapist might yearn to fulfill.

Beginning art therapists, still treading unfamiliar ground, may feel surer of foot shod with well-worn assessment procedures developed by senior art therapists. For example, many a time I have assigned students to practice conducting an assessment interview, encouraging them to develop a series of art tasks that would provide the information they are seeking, only to have them respond with, "I have decided to do the Ulman" (a much used series developed by Elinor Ulman). Questions of validity and reliability of the test are seldom raised.

Although in the broadest sense of the word, assessment is a continuous part of a psychotherapist's ongoing work in monitoring a client's progress, in its more specific usage assessment is a procedure for gathering information about the client. The information may include both history and present state. There are various purposes for conducting an art therapy assessment (Wadeson, 1989). The most common is an initial interview for treatment planning. This may include a determination of whether art therapy would be beneficial to the client. Under these circumstances, establishment of rapport would be an important ingredient in the assessment session. In treatment planning, information revealed in an art assessment may open doors to significant passages for work. For example, a psychiatrist and social worker working with a hospitalized depressed man and his wife felt stuck in their therapy with the couple because the husband was so withdrawn. In desperation, they requested an art therapy assessment session which they observed through a two-way mirror.

One of the pictures that I requested the couple each draw was an abstract of their marital relationship (Wadeson, 1980). The husband drew an enclosed form and said he felt trapped. After the session, the psychiatrist said he learned more about the couple than he had in ten verbal sessions. From observing only one art therapy assessment, the psychiatrist and social worker were able to continue verbal couple therapy, now no longer stuck.

When I worked at the National Institute of Mental Health where research projects required cohorts of a specific diagnosis, if researchers had doubts, they often looked to art therapy assessment for more specific information. Sometimes the art provided it. For example, although it appeared that the previous delusional state of a newly admitted schizophrenic patient had cleared, the art therapy assessment revealed delusional ideation.

In addition to diagnosis and current mental state, other specific information may be sought, for example, suicide risk or previous sexual abuse. Obviously these are important issues in treatment.

Assessment may be used for research as well. In such, the art may serve as a barometer, as in noting responses to medication, for example (Wadeson and Epstein, 1975). Or the art itself may be the subject of investigation as in noting the characteristics of art expression in depression (Wadeson, 1971).

Although the examples above illustrate the fertile possibilities of information that art expression can provide, art images are like dreams in their illusiveness. There is no dictionary of meanings that can be applied to either. And there remains enormous confusion, both on the part of art therapists and those who work with them, as to just what can be gleaned from art therapy assessments. One can readily note artistic style, such as disorganization, emptiness, or intensity of color. But does it tell us the client is disorganized, empty, or intense? Content can be even more puzzling. Unless the client tells us, do we know that the house he has drawn is his childhood home, a symbol for himself, a stereotyped image he drew as a child? Is it possible to determine either suicide risk or sexual abuse from art? Sometimes. Can you count on it? No. Do some art therapists and their colleagues believe otherwise? Yes.

Into this murky realm of uncertainty, misinformation, and confusion, Stephanie Brooke shines a beacon of clarity. She has selected a variety of frequently used art therapy assessment instruments for review. Her evaluations of them that she has compiled in this book are a significant contribution to the field in several different ways. Most immediately, they do provide "tools of the trade" with clear presentations of the information necessary for each test, including specifics such as authors, publishers, costs, time limits for administration, and so forth. A thorough discussion follows covering test purpose, dimensions to be measured, administration, norm groups, score interpretation, validity and reliability measurements, and related research including utilization with various populations. Unique in art therapy literature is Stephanie Brooke's evaluation of each test for both desirable and undesirable features and an overall evaluation that shows clearly just what the test can and cannot do. In some instances, test authors have made claims that Brooke has discovered to be unsound. The analysis of each test is both thorough and concise, well organized, and clearly presented. Armed with this information, the art therapist knows exactly what to expect from each procedure.

The tests the author has chosen to review a broad range of assessment questions, including pathology, cognition, family dynamics, multicultural issues, self-perception, spiritual and relationship issues. After discussing each assessment procedure, she summarizes all their strengths and weaknesses. The book concludes with a recommendation to evaluate a client by utilizing a combination of assessments. A case study provides an example of how this may be done and the information that may be gained.

In addition to supplying "tools of the trade," this book provides a significant picture of the state of the art in art therapy assessment. Stephanie Brooke shows us how far we have come and how far we need to go in designing art therapy assessment instruments.

Harriet Wadeson, Ph.D., A.T.R.-BC, HLM

References

Wadeson, H. (1980), *Art Psychotherapy*, John Wiley, New York.

Wadeson, H. (1989), *The Dynamics of Art Psychotherapy*, John Wiley, New York.

Wadeson, H. (1971), Characteristics of Art Expression in Depression, *Journal of Nervous and Mental Disease*, 153 (3).

Wadeson, H., and Epstein, R., (1975) Intrapsychic Effect of Amphetamine in Hyperkinesis as Revealed Through Art Productions, *Psychiatry and Art*, S. Karger, Basel.

PREFACE

When I was in graduate school studying to be a counselor, I heard several of my peers talking about "Tests and Measurements." It was one of the core courses for my tract in Community Agency Counseling. Often, I would hear my colleagues say, "You will hate that course," "Bite the bullet and just try and get through it," and "I had a 4.0 until that course." Needless to say, I was very anxious about taking "Tests and Measurements." Worse yet, I was taking it as a summer course. Granted, the math part of the course was challenging at times, yet the most interesting part was writing the final paper. Part of the class requirements included writing a complete test review. We were expected to pick out an assessment and then critique it according to the *Standards for Educational and Psychological Testing* (AERA, APA, NCME, 1985). Although an overwhelming task at first, I found that I was able to apply the information from class in a way that was meaningful to me. Fortunately, I had a wonderful professor who taught the class to write a test review in an organized, coherent, and logical fashion. In addition, the format that he gave us was that which professional journals, such as *Measurement and Evaluation in Counseling and Development,* expect. Thus, I wrote my first test review that was later accepted for publication (Brooke, 1993).

This course influenced me in that I continued writing test reviews after graduation. As a counselor, I feel a responsibility to my clients with respect to the assessments that I administer. I want to know if the test is reliable and valid. If that information is not available, I want to know what information that the test will yield. Prior to giving an assessment, I first made sure that it was necessary and beneficial to the client in the type of information it provided. Second, I researched the test manual. How closely did the test manual follow educational and psychological testing standards? Was it reliable? More importantly, was the test valid? What information would this test yield that might promote client growth and development? These were just a few of the questions that I considered.

As a private therapist, I often used art therapy techniques when working with my clients. I specialized in sexual abuse issues; therefore, I was drawn to a therapeutic mode that was nonthreatening. For my clients, art was a powerful mode through which they expressed their feelings, thoughts, fears, and wishes. Qualitatively and quantitatively, I saw improvement in self-esteem. Art seemed to be a natural, non-threatening method for dealing with sexual abuse issues. Since that time, I have never taken for granted the healing power of art. I agree with McNiff (1992) in that art is "a medicine that proceeds through different phases of creation and reflection. Although therapists and other people involved in this process make their contributions as guides and witnesses, the medicinal agent is art itself, which releases and contains psyche's therapeutic forces." (p. 3)

The purpose of this book is to provide counselors and therapists, who use art as an adjunct therapy or primary therapy, with reviews of traditional and current art therapy assessments. It is beyond the scope of this book to include all art therapy assessments. The tests reviewed will be useful to clinicians specializing in a variety of areas: family, cross-cultural, spiritual, and individual counseling. Since only a few art therapy assessments are standardized, such as the Silver Drawing Test (1990) and the Diagnostic Drawing Series (Cohen, 1985), the remainder of the assessments will be reviewed on the research conducted to date and the type of information that the test yields.

Chapter 1 presents an introduction to art therapy and the process of assessment. Chapters 2 through 12 consider several art therapy assessments, beginning with traditional tests and ending with current releases. Validity, reliability, research using the assessment, and the type of clinical information the assessment yields are considered. Chapter 13 presents recommendations for the various assessments based upon the strengths and weaknesses of the approach. The last chapter involves a case study that demonstrates how several art therapy assessments can be used to provide a more complete clinical profile of a client.

ACKNOWLEDGMENTS

There are many individuals that I would like to express my appreciation to in the completion of this work. First, I am grateful to Dr. Jack Dilendik, my former advisor, for his friendship, support, and inspiration in my writing ventures. I would like to thank Dr. Joseph Ciechalski, who continually provided encouragement for my professional endeavors. Also, I am indebted to Joe and Ellen Darby, MA, ATR, for their reflective comments regarding this manuscript. To Dr. Deana Morrow, I would like to express my deep appreciation for her support and resourcefulness regarding my private practice. I am thankful to Gary Cvejic, my best friend, who worked patiently with me on the photographs and typesetting. I am also grateful to Martin Johnson who provided valuable suggestions regarding the art work for this book. Finally, I would like to thank Marty and Cindy Pearson, two of my oldest and closest friends, for their strength and inspiration.

CONTENTS

A THERAPIST'S GUIDE TO
ART THERAPY ASSESSMENTS

Chapter 1

INTRODUCTION TO ART THERAPY ASSESSMENT

THE USE OF ART IN THERAPY:

Due to the increasing isolation, dehumanization, and overintellectualization of our culture, there is an increasing focus on affect and getting in touch with the inner self (Moreno, 1975). Accordingly, therapists are inclined to use nonverbal approaches such as art, music, dance, and drama for psychological healing and growth. Although these methods may be unorthodox to some, people can encounter important self-data by approaching themselves from a new perspective or through a new medium.

Art has been used as a means of self-expression for centuries. People have used art materials to "make images and connect them to feelings and bodily states [that] bring into the open thoughts that have been only vaguely sensed" (Keyes, 1983, p. 104). Edwards (1986) asserted that drawing exists as a parallel to verbal language and was the simplest of nonverbal languages. Art does not have the restriction of linguistic development in order to convey thoughts or feelings.

> Aside from the therapeutic benefit of nonverbal communication of thoughts and feelings, one of the most impressive aspects of the art process is its potential to achieve or restore psychological equilibrium. This use of the art process as intervention is not mysterious or particularly novel; it may have been one of the reasons humankind developed art in the first place—to alleviate or contain feelings of trauma, fear, anxiety, and psychological threats to the self and the community. (Malchiodi, 1990, p. 5)

Projective methods designed to explore motivation are not new to the field of psychotherapy. Machover (1949) observed the power of projective methods in discovering unconscious determinants of self-expression that were not apparent in direct, verbal communication. Langer (1953) stressed that "there is an important part of reality that is quite inaccessible to the formative influence of language: that is the realm of the so-called 'inner experience,' the life of feeling and emotion . . . the primary function of art is to objectify feeling so that we can contemplate and understand it" (p. 4–5). Art expression offers the opportunity to explore personal problems without dependence on a verbal mode of communication. Naumburg (1966), a renowned art therapist, contended that "by projecting interior images into exteriorized designs art therapy crystallizes and fixes in lasting form the recollections of dreams of phantasies which would otherwise remain evanescent and might quickly be forgotten" (p. 2). According to Knoff and Prout (1985), projective drawings were used for the following purposes:

1. as an ice-breaker technique to facilitate child-examiner rapport and the child's comfort, trust, and motivation.
2. as a sample of behavior that involves a child's reactions to one-on-one child-examiner interaction with a semi-structured task.
3. as a technique that investigates the interaction between a child's or adolescent's personality and his/her perceptions of relationships among peers, family, school, and significant others.
4. as a technique linked to a clinical, diagnostic interview that moves discussion beyond a drawing's actions and dynamics to more pervasive psychological issues and concerns

Therapists have found that drawings serve as an indication of the client's current level of functioning. Often, drawings are part of an initial interview with a client. Over the years, these techniques have formed the foundation of art therapy assessment. The next section will discuss the use of drawings within the assessment process.

ART THERAPY ASSESSMENTS:

There are many questions regarding the nature and objectives of art therapy assessments. "The purpose of the assessment process is to study an individual's behavior through observation of his/her performance and through a systematic examination of his/her finished product" (Oster & Gould, 1987, p. 13). Art therapy assessments may be viewed as tests of personality. Anastasi (1988) defined personality tests as "measures of such characteristics as emotional states, interpersonal relations, motivations, interests, and attitudes" (p. 17). Generally, there are three types of personality assessments: self-report inventories, performance tests, and projective techniques. Art therapy assessments may be considered the latter type. Anastasi (1988) defined projective techniques as tests in which "the client is given a relatively unstructured task that permits wide latitude in its solution. The assumption underlying such methods is that the individual will project her or his characteristic modes of response into such a task" (p. 19). These tests are disguised in their purpose, somewhat similar to the performance tests. This reduces the likelihood that the client will "fake" or generate a desired response. The purpose of this book is to discuss the advantages and disadvantages of the various art therapy assessments. As Anastasi (1988) noted:

> Research on the measurement of personality has attained impressive proportions since 1950, and many igneous devices and technical improvements are under investigation. It is rather the special difficulties encountered in the measurement of personality that account for the slow advances in this area. (p. 19)

SCOPE OF ART THERAPY ASSESSMENTS:

An area of controversy concerning projective assessments centered on validity and reliability. "The psychologist trained in research design and statistics, sought to demonstrate the validity and reliability of projective drawings, while chief interest of the therapists (who had no training in research) was in how art could contribute to understanding individual patients and therefore, might assist in developing therapeutic technique" (Wadeson, 1992, p. 136). Some psychologists stated that projective drawing techniques were not valid indications of personality traits (Swenson, 1957, 1968; Klopfer & Taulbee, 1976; Chapman & Chapman, 1967, 1969, and Wanderer, 1969). Despite these findings, researchers still use projective drawings for diagnosis and treatment. Groth-Marant (1990) provided evidence of validity and reliability with respect to projective drawings. The question of validity is still being debated today.

Controversy also focused on structured drawing tasks and spontaneous drawings. Often there is overlap, as Naumburg (1953, p. 124) observed:

> The line of demarcation between studies . . . that employ spontaneous art as a primary means of psychotherapy and those that deal mainly with structured art in diagnosis is not always easy to define. In some cases the therapeutic approach that uses spontaneous art may also include more formal diagnostic art elements; similarly structured art tests may include elements free of art expression as employed in art therapy. An example of this overlapping of areas of therapy and diagnosis is evident in those diagnostic papers which discuss figure and family drawings; in such cases, it can be observed that while the theme for a specific type of figure drawing is set by the therapist, spontaneity is nevertheless encouraged in the execution of this task by the patient.

Since each art therapy assessment has its own value and limitations, this book will include structured as well as unstructured approaches.

Neale and Rosal (1993) reviewed some common projective drawing techniques. These authors noted the value of these techniques as instruments of insight and information that can be utilized across professions. Although the projective techniques have great potential in revealing personality characteristics, there were several questions that the authors had (p. 37):

- how accurate is the diagnostic information taken from drawings and paintings?
- should strengths as well as weaknesses be sought in drawings?
- can drawings be used to assess pathology?
- how sensitive are drawings to clinical and therapeutic changes?
- should drawings and paintings be used to assess pathology and to diagnose?

These are questions typically asked by psychologists who use projective techniques. Art therapy assessments are sometimes designed differently from the projective techniques created by psychologists. Neale and Rosal (1993) outlined some concerns that art therapists have regarding assessments (p. 38):

- can objective drawing characteristics be identified without losing the holistic view of the drawing?
- can diagnostic indicators be identified?
- can diagnosis be reached through one drawing?
- how is a scoring manual developed?
- can free drawings as well as set drawing tasks be used in diagnosis and how does one score a free drawing?

These are just a few of the questions that will be considered in this book. Where applicable, I will critique reliability and validity information. If that data is not present for a particular assessment, information that the test purports to yield will be considered.

Another factor that will be deliberated is the cookbook approach to art therapy assessment:

> In the "cookbook" method you look up the meaning of each sign and come up with a ready made diagnosis without regard for the total figure drawn and irrespective of the child's age, sex, intelligence, and social-cultural background. The circumstance under which the drawing was produced are also ignored. (Koppitz, 1968, p. 55)

There are obvious disadvantages to looking up the meaning of images in a dictionary fashion. Images have various meanings to different individuals. Additionally, observation of the client while completing the assessment provides valuable information about affect and personality. Despite the limitations discussed, art therapy assessments are a valuable source for understanding client issues and dynamics. Although many assessments in this book do not yield quantitative information, they provide a rich source of client information:

> Even without this quantification, clinicians are holding firm to the belief that drawings can be considered a unique, personal expression of inner experiences which, when used appropriately, can offer clues that are of value both diagnostically and therapeutically. Even though the value of drawings cannot be measured independently from the accumulated knowledge of the clinician, this does not diminish their intrinsic value as aids in working with both impaired and growth-oriented populations. (Oster & Gould, 1987, p. 8)

The book will begin with some traditional art therapy assessments and then proceed to more recent measures. It should be noted that the assessments reviewed in this book represent those more commonly used in graduate programs, private practices, and clinical settings. Chapter 13 presents a summary of the previous chapters as well as my recommendations for the art therapy assessments reviewed. Chapter 14 provides the reader with a method for using and writing the results of art therapy assessments.

REFERENCES

Anastasi, A. (1988). *Psychological testing.* 6th ed. New York: Macmillian.

Chapman, L., and Chapman, J. (1967). Genesis of popular but erroneous psychodiagnostic observations. *Journal of Abnormal Psychology, 72,* 193–204.

Chapman, L., and Chapman, J. (1969). Illusory correlation as an obstacle to the use of valid psychodiagnostic signs. *Journal of Abnormal Psychology, 74,* 271–280.

Edwards, B. (1986). *Drawing on the artist within.* New York: Simon and Schuster.

Groth-Marant, G. (1990). *Handbook of psychological assessment.* (2nd ed.) New York: John Wiley & Sons.

Keyes, M.F. (1983). *Inward journey: Art as therapy.* Lasalle, IL: Open Court.

Klopfer, W., and Taulbee, E. (1976). Projective tests. In: M. Rosenzweig & L. Porter, Eds. *Annual Review of Psychology, 27.* Palo Alto, CA: Annual Reviews Inc.

Knoff, H.M., and Prout, H.T. (1985). The kinetic drawing system: A review and integration of the Kinetic Family and School Drawing techniques. *Psychology in the Schools, 22 (January),* 50–59.

Koppitz, E.M. (1968). *Psychological evaluation of children's human figure drawings.* New York: Grune & Stratton.

Langer, S. (1953). *Feeling and Form.* New York: Charles Schribner's Sons.

Machover, K. (1949). *Personality projection in the drawing of the human figure.* Springfield, IL: Charles C Thomas.

Malchiodi, C.A. (1990). *Breaking the silence: Art therapy with children from violent homes.* New York: Brunner/Mazel.

Moreno, Z.T. (1975). *Group psychotherapy and psychodrama.* New York: Beacon House.

Naumburg, M. (1953). *Psychoneurotic art: Its function in psychotherapy.* New York: Grune & Stratton.

Naumburg, M. (1966). *Dynamically oriented art therapy.* New York: Grune & Stratton.

Neale, E.L., and Rosal, M.L. (1993). What can art therapists learn from the research on projective drawing techniques for children? A review of the literature. *The Arts in Psychotherapy, 20,* 37–49.

Oster, G.D., and Gould, P. (1987). *Using drawings in assessment and therapy: A guide for mental health professionals.* New York: Brunner/Mazel.

Silver, R. (1990). *Silver Drawing Test of Cognitive Skills and Adjustment.* Sarasota, FL: Ablin Press.

Swenson, C. (1957). Empirical evaluations of human figure drawings. *Psychological Bulletin, 54,* 431–466.

Swenson, C. (1968). Empirical evaluations of human figure drawings: 1957–1966. *Psychological Bulletin, 70,* 20–44.

Wadeson, H. ed. (1992). *A guide to conducting art therapy research.* Mundelein, IL: The American Art Therapy Association.

Wanderer, Z. (1969). Validity of clinical judgments based on human figure drawings. *Journal of Consulting and Clinical Psychology, 33,* 143–150.

Chapter 2

HUMAN FIGURE DRAWING TEST

TITLE: Human Figure Drawing Test (HFD)

AGE: ages five to twelve

YEAR: 1968

PURPOSE: designed to determine developmental level as well as provide information on personality characteristics

SCORES: two scores: (1) developmental items Present (total of 30 points) and (2) emotional indicators Present (total of 30 points)

MANUAL: manual (341 pages); illustrations (111 pages); profile (4 pages); reliability data (1 page); validity data (44 pages)

TIME LIMIT: no time limit for administration

COST: $71.95 for testing manual

AUTHOR: Koppitz, Elizabeth M.

PUBLISHER: Grune & Stratton Inc., 111 Fifth Avenue, New York, NY, 10003.

INTRODUCTION

Some Human Figure Drawing (HFD) tests focused on emotional indicators while ignoring or minimizing the developmental aspects of a drawing. Other HFD tests considered only developmental signs and neglected emotional indicators. Some test developers viewed items as a measure of both development and personality characteristics. Due to the confusion of previous human figure drawing tests, Koppitz (1968) designed the HFD to include separate indices of development and personality characteristics. For example, the omission of the neck or feet on HFDs was not uncommon for normal five-year-old boys, developmentally speaking. Yet by the age of ten, boys should be including these features in their drawing, the omission of which may indicate immaturity or emotional problems. "It appears, therefore, that a meaningful interpretation of HFDs of children presupposes a thorough knowledge of both developmental and emotional indicators on drawings at each age level and a clear differentiation between the two" (Koppitz, 1968, p. 3).

Koppitz (1968) systematically investigated the HFDs of children rang-ing in age from five to twelve. Her intention was to redesign the assessment so that it served as a development test and as a projective test.

PURPOSE AND RECOMMENDED USE:

The HFD was the product of an interpersonal situation in which the clinician asked the child to draw a whole person. The structure of the drawing was said to indicate the child's maturational level, whereas the style indicated the child's attitudes. The HFD may serve as a self-portrait, a picture of the client's inner self and his attitudes. Only one drawing was required to yield clinical information about a child. The HFD was designed for psychologists who work in clinics, schools, hospitals, or in private practice.

DIMENSIONS THAT THE TEST PURPORTS TO MEASURE:

The HFD measured a child's developmental level and attitude. The first measure, developmental items, included 30 features of human figures. Specifically, a developmental item was defined "as an item that occurs only on relatively few HFDs of children of a younger age level and then increases in frequency of occurrence as the age of the children increases, until it gets to be a regular feature of many or most HFDs at a given age level" (Koppitz, 1968, p. 9). The presence of these items was related to the child's maturational level not to his/her artistic ability, school learning, or medium used.

The second dimension that the HFD purported to measure was emotional indicators. An emotional indicator was defined "as a sign on HFDs which meets the following three criteria:

(1) It must have clinical validity, i.e., it must be able to differentiate between HFDs of children with and without emotional problems.
(2) It must be unusual and occur infrequently on the HFDs of normal children who are not psychiatric patients, i.e., the sign must be present on less than 16 percent of the HFDs of children at a given age level.
(3) It must not be related to age and maturation, i.e., its frequency of

occurrence on HFDs must not increase solely on the basis of the children's increase in age" (Koppitz, 1968, p. 35).

Thirty-eight items were selected. The indicators measured the quality of the drawing, unusual features, and characteristic omissions of children at a given age level. Out of 38 original items, 30 met the criteria as outlined by Koppitz (1968).

ADMINISTRATION:

The HFD can be administered individually or in group settings. Koppitz (1968) recommended individual testing since the administrator was able to observe the child and ask questions if needed. Also, "most children produce richer and more revealing drawings in a one-to-one relationship with an accepting psychologist than in a group setting" (Koppitz, 1968, p. 6).

The HFD utilized a blank sheet of white paper size 8 1/2″ by 11″ with a number two pencil and eraser. The following directions were given:

> On this piece of paper, I would like you to draw a WHOLE person. It can be any kind of a person you want to draw, just make sure that it is a whole person and not a stick figure or a cartoon figure. (Koppitz, 1968, p. 6)

There was no time limit for the administration of the HFD. Generally, children took 10 to 30 minutes to complete the assessment. The child was permitted to erase as needed. Koppitz (1968) instructed that the examiner should carefully observe the child to determine the sequence in which the figure was completed, affect, spontaneous comments, and behavioral changes.

In order to avoid copying, children should be seated as far apart as possible when administering the HFD to a group. When tested individually, the child should be seated in a manner that he/she does not see a picture of a person on a wall or on a magazine cover. Using the examiner as a model for the assessment should be discouraged. If a child was inclined to copy figures, the examiner should repeat the HFD with the added instruction to draw "a picture of a whole person out of your own head" (Koppitz, 1968, p. 7).

NORM GROUPS:

The normative sample included 1856 public school children from kindergarten through sixth grade. The sample contained students from ten different schools. One-third of the students came from low income communities (including black and white students), one-third came from a white, middle income community, and the last one-third lived in high income areas. Other demographic characteristics of the sample were not discussed. Additionally, it did not appear to be a random sample. Koppitz (1968) provided a breakdown of the sample by age and gender. In her opinion, the sample did not include children who were mentally retarded or physically handicapped. The students were given the HFD in a group format by their teacher. Koppitz (1968) checked the HFDs for the presence of the 30 developmental items and the 30 emotional indicators.

INTERPRETATION OF SCORES:

For the developmental items, charts were provided to aid in the interpretation of scores. For example, if a child had an HFD score of seven or eight, his level of mental ability was rated as high average to superior (IQ 110 upward). If a child had an HFD score of one or zero, he was rated as mentally retarded (IQ less than 70). Charts were not provided for the emotional indicators; therefore, quantitative interpretation of this section of the test was not possible. Qualitative interpretation focused on how the child drew the figure, who the figure represented, and the child's verbalizations. Koppitz (1968) interpreted HFDs based on the following: (1) the child's approach toward life's problems; (2) attitudes toward significant events; and (3) attitude toward self. Her interpretations were supported by case studies. For instance, three of her cases approached life problems with ambitious attitudes. These children drew themselves climbing mountains.

SOURCE OF ITEMS:

The developmental items were taken from the Goodenough-Harris (Harris, 1963) scoring system and Koppitz' own experience. Only items that pertained to elementary age school children were included. The developmental items were broken down into the following categories: (1)

Expected items (occur on 86–100% of drawings); (2) Common items (occur in 51–85% of HFDs); (3) Not unusual items (occur in 16–50% of drawings); and (4) Exceptional items (occur in 15% or less of drawings). Koppitz (1968) then broke down the scores by gender and age. She indicated which features were expected, common, not unusual, and exceptional. For instance, a five-year-old boy can be expected to include six basic items on their HFDs: head, eyes, nose, mouth, body, and legs. It was exceptional for a five-year-old boy to draw pupils, two dimensional feet, correct number of digits, arms at shoulder, nostrils, lips, and knees. Five-year-old girls were expected to include seven items on their HFDs: head, eyes, nose, mouth, body, legs, and arms. It was exceptional for five-year-old girls to draw nostrils, elbows, lips, arms at shoulders, and knees.

Emotional indicators were broken down by age and gender. Two criteria were used: (1) that the item was not related to child's developmental level and (2) that the item was unusual and occurred in less that 15 percent of the sample. Eight items of the original sample of 38 did not meet the criteria; therefore, they were omitted from the assessment. For instance, 15 percent of the six-year-old children (N = 131) showed poor integration of their figure. For six-year-old girls (N = 133), 8 percent showed poor integration of their figure.

VALIDITY AS DETERMINED BY THE AUTHOR:

Validity of Developmental Items

To determine the validity of the developmental items on the HFD, Koppitz (1966) examined 45 boys and 49 girls who were attending kindergarten classes. She wanted to see if the drawing medium had an effect on the HFD. The children were administered the test individually. Koppitz (1966) observed behavioral differences between boys and girls. Boys were awkward, shy, and seemed inept at using the No. 2 pencil. On the other hand, girls appeared comfortable and at ease using a No. 2 pencil. A few weeks later, the classroom teachers administered the HFD in a group fashion, modifying the instructions. Children were instructed to use crayons and were given the following directions:

Now that you are going into the first grade, I would like to have a picture of you to keep. So make me a picture of what you look like. Do not look at anyone else's paper because no two boys and girls look alike. (Koppitz, 1968, p. 21)

It should be noted that these instructions differ from the original HFD directive. No time limit was set. All pencil drawings and crayon drawings were checked for the presence of developmental items. Some items were omitted since the children were so young (i.e., two lips, elbow, knee, profile, good proportion, two or more clothing items). Using percentage of children who revealed the developmental items, Koppitz (1966) found "thirteen basic items on HFDs were truly developmental indicators for young children and were not much influenced by the drawing medium or by the instructions given to the children" (p. 22). Overall, girls used pencil better than boys whereas boys were more proficient using crayons. She did find that children were more likely to draw hair and clothing more often when using crayons as compared to pencil. It was unclear if these were significant differences.

The effect of learning and maturation on HFDs was examined using 179 children (89 boys and 90 girls) attending kindergarten classes. Koppitz (1968) compared the HFDs of children, matched by age, who either did or did not have a year of kindergarten training. The test was administered at the beginning of the school year in a group fashion and then again, nine months later. The drawings were scored for the presence of the 23 developmental items. By the end of the school year, 20 of the 23 developmental items were found more often than in the beginning of the year. Since it was difficult to discern if the improvement on the HFDs was due to maturation or kindergarten training, Koppitz (1968) matched the HFDs of 35 children (16 pairs of boys and 19 pairs of girls). One set of HFDs came from 35 children who were the oldest students at the beginning of the school year. The other set came from a group of children who were the youngest students prior to beginning school. When comparing these groups, there was very little difference in the frequency of the developmental items. Learning appeared to be related to the presence of the following developmental items: two dimensions on arms and legs, two or more pieces of clothing, and the correct number of fingers. "None of the other 19 developmental items showed a marked increase in frequency of occurrence as the result of school learning, thus supporting the hypothesis that the basic developmental items are primarily related to maturation and are not greatly influenced by school learning" (Koppitz, 1968, p. 26).

To determine the influence of high and low performance ability on HFDs, Koppitz (1968) matched 24 pairs of children by age, gender, and WISC Full Scale IQ (Wechsler, 1949) scores. All the children participating in the study had been referred to the school psychologist for possible learning problems. They ranged in age from 6 to 12 years with a mean age of 10.5 years. One set of the 24 students had a WISC Performance IQ score ten points above their Verbal IQ score. The other set of children had Verbal IQ score that was ten points above their Performance IQ score. Being blind to which group the children belonged to, Koppitz (1968) scored the drawings for the presence of the 30 developmental items. Thereafter, students with high Performance IQ scores were compared to children with low Performance IQ scores. Since the results were not significant, Koppitz (1968) concluded that developmental items on HFDs were not influenced by performance ability; rather, they were related to age and maturation.

In order to learn the relationship between IQ scores and the presence of expected and exceptional items on HFDs, Koppitz (1967) developed a scoring method. Each Expected or Exceptional Item was given a score of $(+1)$ and the omission of an item was given a score of (-1). To avoid negative scores, $(+5)$ points was added to each item whether positively or negatively scored. For example, the omission of one Expected item was given a score of $4 [-1 +5]$. On the other hand, the presence of one Exceptional item was scored as $6 [+1 +5]$. This scoring system was applied to the HFDs of 347 children, ranging in age from 5 to 12 years. The children were evaluated by Koppitz (1967) for psychological difficulties, at which time the HFD was administered. Within one year of the HFD test, the WISC (Wechsler, 1949) or the Standford-Binet Intelligence Scale (Terman and Merril, 1960) was administered to the subjects. Although the subjects showed a wide range of learning difficulties, none was brain injured or suffered from gross physical disabilities. The drawings were scored for the presence of the Expected and Exceptional items and then correlated with the child's IQ score. At the .01 level of significance, Koppitz (1967) found that the child's HFD score correlated with his IQ score. She concluded that the HFD can be used as a rough screening device to assess a child's mental maturity.

Validity of Emotional Indicators

Koppitz examined the validity of the emotional indicators using a sample that included 76 pairs of public school children matched for age and gender. These children were matched with 76 patients in a child guidance clinic, who demonstrated at least normal intelligence. The students were administered the HFD individually. Koppitz found that twelve emotional indicators were found significantly more often in the clinical group than on the drawings of the well-adjusted students. The most significant items (.01 level) included poor integration, shading of body and/or limbs, slanting figure, and tiny figure. The indicators such as the sun and figure cut off by the page were deleted since they did not demonstrate clinical validity.

Next, Koppitz selected 114 psychiatric patients (82 boys and 32 girls) who displayed any one of the following behaviors: overt aggressiveness, extreme shyness (depression or withdrawal), neurotic stealing, or a history of psychosomatic complaints. They ranged in age from 5 to 12 years. None of the children had an IQ score below 70. Shy children were matched with aggressive children. The HFDs were administered individually and checked for the presence of the 30 emotional indicators. Koppitz found that shy children significantly drew tiny figures; omitted the mouth, nose, and eyes more frequently; and showed more hands cut off than did aggressive children. Genitals and transparencies occurred more often in the HFDs of aggressive children. Koppitz warned that no one emotional indicator could distinguish between a shy or aggressive child. Rather, the indicators must be viewed holistically.

Koppitz then compared the HFDs of children who steal with those who had a history of psychosomatic complaints. Few significant differences were found. Koppitz did find that the children with psychosomatic complaints revealed more short arms, legs pressed together, omission of nose and mouth, and clouds. Children who had a history of stealing revealed more shading of hands and/or neck; tiny head; big hands; omission of body, arms, or neck. The omission of the neck was significant at the .01 level.

Koppitz examined the relationship between emotional indicators on HFDs and school achievement. Ranging in age from 5 to 10 years, 313 children (180 rated as good students and 133 as poor students) participated in the study. Using group administration, the HFD was given at the beginning of the school year. The Metropolitan Achievement Test

(Hildreth, 1946) was given at the end of the year and was used to determine the achievement level of the students in the first and second grades. Thereafter, teacher ratings were used. For kindergarten students, the omission of the body and of the mouth distinguished good from poor students. Additionally, 12 of the 13 poor students showed two or more emotional indicators on their HFD compared to three of 13 good pupils. For first and second grade students, five emotional indicators (poor integration, slanting figure, omission of the body and arms, and three or more figures spontaneously drawn) distinguished between good and poor students. For the third and fourth grades, none of the 30 emotional indicators was able to differentiate between the HFDs of good and poor students.

RELIABILITY AS DETERMINED BY THE AUTHOR:

Reliability of the developmental items and for emotional indicators was determined with the aid of another psychologist. Independently, Koppitz (1968) and the psychologist scored HFDs of ten randomly selected second graders. Also, they rated 15 HFDs completed by students referred because of learning and emotional problems. The drawings were checked for the presence of the 30 developmental items and 30 emotional indicators. The examiners reached 95 percent agreement on scoring.

RESEARCH USING THE HFD:

Lingren (1971) attempted to replicate Koppitz' (1968) work with shy and aggressive children. Subjects included 97 pairs of children (56 pairs of boys and 41 pairs of girls) matched by age, gender, and IQ. Children ranged in age from 5 to 12 years. Parents and teachers completed a behavioral checklist that was used to classify the children as shy or aggressive. Children completed the HFD individually. Drawings were scored by Lingren (1971) and a school psychologist for the 30 emotional indicators. They reached 91 percent agreement. Lingren's (1971) results conflicted with Koppitz' findings in that shy children were more likely to draw cut off hands than aggressive children. Lingren (1971) concluded that the 30 emotional indicators could not significantly distinguish shy children from aggressive children. Lingren's work was supported by Hammer and Kaplan (1966) who found that the HFD was not a reliable test. Hammer and Kaplan (1966) had a large sample, 1305 students who were given the HFD and then retested one week later.

Norford and Barakat (1990) also used the HFD to examine possible differences between aggressive and nonaggressive children. The sample ranged in age from four to five years and included 16 aggressive children and 16 nonaggressive children. Aggression was determined by using teacher ratings. Ten clinical raters classified the drawings into two groups: aggressive and nonaggressive. The researchers concluded that the HFD was not a valid instrument for distinguishing between aggressive and nonaggressive students. The authors attributed their findings to the fact that preschool age children lack cognitive maturity and visual-motor coordination.

Cates (1991) compared HFDs of hearing impaired children with normally hearing children. Subjects included 26 residential students at a public school for hearing impaired children. These subjects were matched by age and gender with 26 students in a community school corporation, ranging in age from 9 to 18 years. A diagnosis of profound hearing impairment, placement at the school for at least one year, and a minimum IQ of 80 were the requirements for the hearing impaired sample. For the normally hearing children, the following criteria were used: placement in a regular classroom setting, no history of special education, hearing within a normal range, and no disabling condition. Cates (1991) used the Goodenough-Harris Drawing Test (Harris, 1963) and Koppitz' (1968) emotional indicators. Children were instructed as follows: "I want you to draw a person—the very best person you can. Cartoon characters and stick figures don't count" (Cates, 1991, p. 33). Hearing impaired children were given instructions using American Sign Language (ASL). After completing the drawing, subjects were instructed to identify the sex of the person by writing it at the top of the page. Subjects who drew opposite sex figures were excluded. Drawings were evaluated using emotional indicators (EI) and the Goodenough-Harris (GH) scoring system for drawing of a male or female. Ten drawings were randomly selected, five from the hearing group and five from the hearing impaired group. Although Cates (1991) did not discuss the rater qualifications or the number of raters used, he reported reliability coefficients of .87 for the GH scoring system and .94 for the EI's. He did not find that hearing impaired children drew larger ears than normally hearing individuals, a point supported by Davis and Hoppes (1975). Cates (1991) found a significant correlation of omissions with age and GH scores that suggests that these items may be testing development rather than emotional indices. "Although the results support the comparability of projective drawings between people with a hearing impairment and those with normal hearing, the emotional indicators did not perform as predicted in determining emotional disturbance" (Cates, 1991, p. 33). He went on to question the validity of the emotional indicators. Cates (1991) admitted that the results of his study may not generalize to other samples due to the small sample size and the inability to control for emotional disturbance.

Johnson (1989) examined 32 hearing impaired boys ranging in age from 7 to 12 years attending residential facilities for the deaf. The IQ scores ranged from 70 to 131 with a mean of 106.8. Students were administered the HFD (Koppitz, 1968) and the Stress Response Scales (SRS: Chandler, 1986). Johnson (1989) found that the HFD showed a positive correlation with emotional status as indicated by the SRS. The HFD was highly sensitive to the impulsive and passive-aggressive modes of the SRS. Although he did not use a random sample nor a large sample, Johnson's (1989) work did provide moderate concurrent validity evidence for the HFD (Koppitz, 1968).

Black (1976) randomly selected 100 children ranging in age from 6 to 12 years who were identified as having learning disabilities. Other demographic characteristics of the sample were not discussed such as economic, educational, and religious background. How the children were diagnosed and the nature of the learning disabilities were not discussed. He looked at self-perceived height, actual height, and HFD height discrepancies. Black (1976) concluded that the HFD was an indicator of learning disabilities since he found a significant difference in the mean actual height and the mean estimated height. Younger children were highly inaccurate when estimating height. Also, females were significantly more accurate in estimating their height as compared to males. Since there was not a significant number of drawings where height was scored as either large or small, Black (1976) asserted that the HFD may not be a direct representation of body image. Neal and Rosal (1993) supported Black (1976) in that the height of the HFD may not be a reliable indicator particularly for learning disabilities.

Glutting and Nester (1986) examined the HFDs of 161 kindergarten children (82 males, 79 females). Using two learning related behavior tests, the researchers wanted to examine the predictability of the HFD. Children were placed into one of three groups depending on the number of emotional indicators present: (1) well adjusted (no EIs); (2) adequately adjusted (one EI); or (3) possibly maladjusted (two or more EIs). Glutting and Nester (1986) found support for the concurrent validity of the HFD in that it significantly distinguished between the three groups of children.

Koppitz and Casullo (1983) examined cultural influences on HFDs. Using two matched groups of 147 Argentine and 147 USA adolescents, the researchers found that the drawings reflected different cultural values. Argentine children were better controlled, less aggressive, more vague and more concerned with appearance and behavior. On the other hand, USA subjects portrayed more outgoing, impulsive, insecure, and aggressive behaviors.

Hibbard and Hartman (1990) examined the discriminant validity of the HFD. Drawings from 65 alleged sexual abuse victims were compared to 64 drawings made by subjects who were presumed not to be victims of sexual abuse. No significant differences were found between the two groups on emotional indicators. As a group, the alleged victims tended to draw some indicators more often: legs pressed together, big hands, and genitals. Additionally, the victim group significantly showed more anxiety than the comparison group. The researchers stressed that the emotional indicators be reevaluated since they were found in the comparison group. It may be that some subjects in the comparison group were survivors of sexual abuse who may not have disclosed the information to the researchers or may not remember the abuse.

DESIRABLE FEATURES:

Koppitz (1968) clearly described each item in the developmental and emotional indicator lists. In addition, she used examples in the case studies to illustrate the items. One chapter included case studies that relate the HFD to mental development, school achievement, organic conditions, and personality characteristics.

UNDESIRABLE FEATURES:

The quantitative scoring procedure for the emotional indicators seems pointless since Koppitz (1968) did not provide guidelines for interpretation. In addition, interpretation may be difficult without previous clinical experience. Koppitz (1968) discussed possible interpretations of HFDs, but they were based on case studies. Quantitative scoring procedures were not demonstrated in the case studies used in the book.

OVERALL EVALUATION:

Koppitz' (1968) HFD did show some discriminant validity, particularly with high achievers compared to low achievers. Although she demonstrated that the HFD can discriminate between shy and aggressive children, other researchers were unable to reach the same conclusion. Discriminant validity for the HFD was lacking. From the research to date, the HFD did not discriminate sexually abused, learning disabled, or aggressive children from "normal" populations. Additional research is needed on the developmental items on the HFD. Motta et al. (1993) argued that the HFD was not a reliable or valid instrument for assessing intelligence. Also, information on the reliability of the HFD needs to be examined. Since the standardization sample was selected over 30 years ago, future research should focus on reestablishing norms for the HFD.

REFERENCES

Black, F.W. (1976). The size of human figure drawings of learning disabled children. *Journal of Clinical Psychology, 32(3)*, 736–741.

Cates, J.A. (1991). Comparison of Human Figure Drawings by hearing and hearing impaired children. *The Volta Review, January*, 31–39.

Chandler, L. (1985). *The Stress Response Scale: A Manual.* Pittsburgh, PA: University of Pittsburgh Psychoeducational Clinic.

Davis, C.J., and Hoppes, J.L. (1975). Comparison of House-Tree-Person drawings of young deaf and hearing children. *Journal of Personality Assessment, 39*, 28–33.

Glutting, J.J., and Nester, A. (1986). Koppitz emotional indicators as predictors of kindergarten children's learning-related behavior. *Contemporary Educational Psychology, 11*, 117–126.

Hammer, M., and Kaplan, A.M. (1966). The reliability of children's human figure drawings. *Journal of Clinical Psychology, 22*, 316–319.

Harris, D.B. (1963). *Children's Drawings as Measures of Intellectual Maturity.* New York: Harcourt, Brace, and World, Inc.

Hibbard, R.A., and Hartman, G.L. (1990). Emotional indicators in human figure drawings of sexually victimized and nonabused children. *Journal of Clinical Psychology, 46(2)*, 211–219.

Hildreth, G. (1946). *Metropolitan Achievement Test, Primary I Battery: Form R.* Yonkerson-Hudson: World Book.

Johnson, G.S. (1989). Emotional Indicators in the Human Figure Drawings of impaired children: A small sample validation study. *AAD, July*, 205–208.

Koppitz, E.M. (1968). *Psychological evaluation of children's human figure drawings.* New York: Grune & Stratton.

Koppitz, E.M. (1967). Expected and exceptional items on Human Figure Drawings and IQ scores of children age 5–12. *Journal of Clinical Psychology, 23,* 81–83.

Koppitz, E.M. (1966). Emotional indicators on Human Figure Drawings of shy and aggressive children. *Journal of Clinical Psychology, 22,* 466–469.

Koppitz, E.M. (1966). Emotional indicators on Human Figure Drawings of children: A validation study. *Journal of Clinical Psychology, 22,* 313–315.

Koppitz, E.M. (1966). Emotional indicators on Human Figure Drawings and school achievement of first and second graders. *Journal of Clinical Psychology, 22,* 481–483.

Koppitz, E.M., and Casullo, M.M. (1983). Exploring cultural influences on human figure drawings of young adolescents. *Perceptual and Motor Skills, 57,* 479–483.

Lingren, R.H. (1971). An attempted replication of emotional indicators in human figure drawings by shy and aggressive children. *Psychological Reports, 29,* 35–38.

Motta, R.W., Little, S.G., and Tobin, M.I. (1993). The use and abuse of human figure drawings. *School Psychology Quarterly, 8(3),* 162–169.

Neale, E.L., and Rosal, M.L. (1993). What can art therapists learn from the research on projective drawing techniques for children? A review of the literature. *The Arts in Psychotherapy, 20,* 37–49.

Norford, B.C., and Barakat, L.P. (1990). The relationship of human figure drawings to aggressive behavior in preschool children. *Psychology in the Schools, 27,* 318–325.

Terman, L.M., and Merrill, M.A. (1960). *Standford-Binet Intelligence Scale.* Boston, MA: Houghton-Mifflin.

Wechsler, D. (1949). *Wechsler Intelligence Scale for Children.* New York, NY: The Psychological Corporation.

Chapter 3

KINETIC FAMILY DRAWINGS

TITLE: Kinetic Family Drawings (KFD)
AGE: age limit not presented
YEAR: 1972
PURPOSE: designed to understand child development: self-concept
                and interpersonal relationships
SCORES: interpretation is based on actions, styles, and symbols
                used in the drawing; scoring is based on using a grid to
                measure distance of the self from other figures and size
                of the figures; an analysis sheet is included that sum-
                marizes information from the grid and drawing charac-
                teristics
MANUAL: manual (304 pages); illustrations (137 pages); profile (2
                pages); reliability data (none reported); validity data
                (none reported)
TIME LIMIT: no time limit for administration
COST: $23.95 for testing manual
AUTHOR: Burns, Robert C., and Kaufman, S.H.
PUBLISHER: Brunner/Mazel, Inc., 19 Union Square, New York, NY,
                10003.

INTRODUCTION:

The Kinetic Family Drawing (KFD) was designed to address the limitations of static family drawings by adding a kinetic component. Burns and Kaufman (1972) asserted that the KFD reflected emotional disturbances faster than interviews or other techniques. The manual was set up in a dictionary fashion so that the reader can look up common actions, styles, and figures in KFDs. Additionally, the manual was filled with example drawings along with case examples. Historical information on the theoretical background and development of the KFD was not discussed.

PURPOSE AND RECOMMENDED USE:

The KFD was developed as a children's assessment to gather information on self-concept and interpersonal relationships. Through the use of the KFD, the therapist can gather information about family dynamics as well as the child's adaptive and defensive functioning. Burns and Kaufman (1970) responded to the feedback given on their previous work, Kinetic Family Drawings, by providing interpretive information about the KFD. A recommended use was not discussed.

DIMENSIONS THAT THE TEST PURPORTS TO MEASURE:

Actions drawn by the client was one dimension that the KFD measured. Action was construed as movement or energy reflected in the various figures (Burns and Kaufman, 1972). For girls, the most frequent actions of the father included reading, cooking, working, burning, mowing, and helping. For boys, the most frequent actions of the father comprised mowing, cutting, reading, repairing, painting, watching television, or working. The percentage of the samples showing these actions were low. For girls, (N = 57) the percentages ranged from seven percent to four percent. For boys (N = 120), the percentages ranged from eight percent to five percent. Similar procedures were used for the actions of the mother and self. Again the percentages were low. According to the authors, girls most frequently drew their mothers cooking, washing dishes, making beds, playing, or vacuuming. Boys, on the other hand, drew their mothers cooking, helping, ironing, planting, vacuuming, sweeping, washing dishes, or sewing. Girls most often drew themselves playing, eating, walking, riding, or washing dishes whereas boys most often drew themselves playing, eating, throwing, riding, or watching television. Movements between figures was also considered. The authors denoted this as a field of force:

> These forces may be conceptualized in a number of ways. Kurt Lewin (1937) might have discussed the drawings in terms of positive and negative valences and various barriers. Freud's (1938) concept of libido, a form of energy, at times invested in a particular person or part of the environment might also be a way to describe the forces depicted in the K-F-D's. Behaviorists, such as B.F. Skinner (1938), might call the emphasized parts of the drawings "discriminative stimuli." (Burns & Kaufman, 1972, p. 46)

The actions were delineated in dictionary fashion including case examples. For instance, the authors began by stating that the most frequent form of an action involved a ball. "Often competition or jealousy is depicted by the path of the ball" (Burns & Kaufman, 1972, p. 54). A great majority of the cases included in this section were devoted to the movement and interpretation of balls. A few other examples of actions were electricity, lights, barriers, fire, and dangerous objects.

Another dimension that the KFD purported to measure was the style of the drawing. Although the authors did not define it, style referred to the way figures were organized on the page and indicated emotional disturbance (Handler & Habenicht, 1994). These styles comprised the following: Compartmentalization, encapsulation, lining at the bottom, underlining figures, edging, lining on the top, and folding compartmentalization. Using a combined sample of 193 children, 20.8 percent had a compartmentalized style of drawing. From the same sample, the lowest figure was 2.1 percent for the use of the folding compartmentalization style. The style categories were vaguely defined. According to the authors, compartmentalization referred to the closing off of one's self or others (Burns and Kaufman, 1972). The examples included figures in boxes. How this differs from encapsulation was not clear. Encapsulated figures were also closed off and in boxes. With respect to encapsulation, the authors stated that "Sometimes we are able to love some people openly, but others bother us, so we encapsulate them" (Burns & Kaufman, 1972, p. 122). Unless the reader was previously familiar with encapsulation and compartmentalization, the distinction between these two styles may be ambiguous. The remainder of the chapter discussed case examples depicting each of the styles outlined by the authors.

The symbols section contained the authors' interpretations of items commonly used on KFDs. Burns and Kaufman (1972) selected a series of recurring symbols to include in this section. For example, the symbol "A" was linked to high academic achievement. The authors reported that it was frequently used in a number of KFD drawings. There was some overlap between symbols and actions in that electricity was listed as a symbol as well as an action; yet, the meaning of electricity in both sections was the same.

The last dimension that the KFD purported to measure was size of figures and the distance between them. The authors created a grid that can be placed over the child's drawing to measure the height of figures as well as the distance of self from other family members. This was a wonderful way to quantify information in the assessment; yet, the authors did not discuss grid analysis in any of the cases presented in the book.

ADMINISTRATION:

The KFD was designed to be an individual assessment. The drawing was completed on plain white paper (8 ½" × 11") using a No. 2 lead pencil. The child was instructed as follows:

> Draw a picture of everyone in your family, including you, DOING something. Try to draw whole people, not cartoons or stick people. Remember, make everyone DOING something—some kind of action. (Burns & Kaufman, 1972, p. 5)

The authors stressed that the examiner should leave the room and check back periodically. No time limit was given. Examiner qualifications were not discussed.

NORM GROUPS:

The actions of individual KFD figures were standardized on a population of 128 males and 65 females ranging in age from 5 to 20 years, with a mean age of 10 years. Although the number of boys outweighed the number of girls, the authors argued that "this ratio is representative of that found by many clinics treating disturbed children" (Burns & Kaufman, 1972, p. 44). With the exception of children completing "normal" KFDs, this sample included cases from their previous book, Kinetic Family Drawings (Burns and Kaufman, 1970). Other demographic characteristics of the sample were not discussed. One was left to believe that the tables in the book were based on a normative sample of emotionally disturbed children. No information was given on how the cases were selected. Moreover, the diagnosis criteria was not described. The population sample was not randomly selected; therefore, the results could not be expected to generalize to other populations.

INTERPRETATION OF SCORES:

A large majority of the book discussed the various symbols, actions, and styles included on the KFD. Some examples were given in the previous section of this chapter, "Dimensions that the The Test Purports to Measure." The authors interpreted the case drawings solely on the basis of drawing style, actions, and symbols. They neglected to use the grid that would have given information about figure sizes and distances between figures. Although the authors created a list of interpretations of common actions, styles, and symbols, they warned that:

> any attempt at hypothesizing the unconscious expression of any single symbol of a dream or projective instrument such as a drawing, one must weigh the alternate and sometimes seemingly incompatible interpretations. What is more essential is that the observer be capable, in the frame of reference of his own background, training and skills, to consider the totality of the individual. (Burns & Kaufman, 1972, p. 144)

The authors did not outline qualifications for administrators nor provide a set of clear guidelines for interpretation. Since the KFD used a dictionary approach and did not observe the drawing process, this method can be classified as a cookbook method (Koppitz, 1968). The authors also created a grid to measure size of figures and distances between them. They did not present guidelines for the interpretation of the measurements. A few questions that came to mind were: How small does a figure have to be to suggest low self-esteem? How far should figures be apart to indicate psychological distance?

SOURCE OF ITEMS:

The source of the symbols, actions, and styles was based on the authors' interpretation of drawings from a sample of children in a clinical setting. Theoretical background and historical development of the KFD were not discussed. No other information on the source of items was presented.

VALIDITY AND RELIABILITY
AS DETERMINED BY THE AUTHOR:

The manual did not discuss validity and reliability data. With the creation of the grid, the authors can feasibly present information on reliability and validity of figure size and distances; yet, this was not done. Also, it should be noted that the information that did appear was based on a biased sample that was not randomly selected. Moreover, it represented a clinical population.

RELIABILITY RESEARCH:

McPhee and Wegner (1976) investigated interrater reliability of the KFD. Using a group of emotionally disturbed children, KFD styles were interpreted. Five judges were trained to score KFDs. Reliability scores ranged from .65 to 1.00 with a median reliability of .87. These scores were in response to compartmentalization, lining at the bottom, and lining at the top drawing styles. The least reliable drawing style was underlining individual figures. Since they occurred very little in their population sample, the authors rejected edging and folding compartmentalization. McPhee and Wegner (1976) also investigated validity of the KFD which will be discussed in the next section of this chapter.

Another study that investigated interrater reliability was completed by Cummings (1980). Two male and two female examiners were trained to score KFDs using three objective scoring methods, one of which was used by McPhee and Wegner (1976). Behavior disordered, learning disabled, and public school children were examined. High interscorer reliabilities resulted. Five weeks later, they retested the children but found that test-retest reliability of the KFDs were inconsistent. Essentially, the KFD could not distinguish between emotionally disturbed children and well adjusted children. Cummings (1980) suggested that the KFD may be sensitive to transition in children's personality states; therefore, it may not be an accurate measure of personality traits or characteristics.

Realizing the lack of an objecting scoring system in the KFD manual, Mostkoff and Lazarus (1983) developed their own system. Fifty elementary school children (25 boys and 25 girls), selected to receive services in reading and math, participated in the study. The group consisted of 14 second grade students, 14 third graders, 9 fourth graders, and 13 fifth graders. Using a two week interval, each child was administered the KFD. The researchers selected 20 variables to interpret the KFDs. Using two raters, interrater reliabilities ranged from .86 to 1.00, with an average reliability of .97. Out of the 20 variables listed by the author, the following revealed significant test-retest reliability: self in picture, omission of body parts (self and others), arm extensions, rotated figures, elevated figures, evasions, barriers, and drawings on the back of the page. "This study shows that it is possible for an objective scoring system to be developed with high interjudge reliability" (Mostkoff & Lazarus, 1983, p. 20). In agreement with Cummings (1980), the authors asserted that the KFD was sensitive to a child's mood changes.

Elin and Nucho (1979) also developed a scoring system for the KFD. Three judges rated 48 KFDs taken from the Burns and Kaufman (1972) manual. They reported high interrater reliability. Additionally, they established concurrent validity using the Personal Adjustment Inventory. The authors argued that the KFD significantly distinguished between low self-esteem and high self-esteem.

Mangold (1982) established that interpretation of the KFD was sensitive to preceding testing conditions. The researcher found that if the KFD was preceded by the Wechsler Intelligence Scale for Children-Revised (WISC–R), it had a suppressing effect on the drawing. If the KFD was preceded by the Rorschach, it had an expanding effect on the drawing. The research was helpful in filtering out extraneous variables that may have affected the interpretation of the KFD.

VALIDITY RESEARCH:

A majority of the studies reviewed in this section did not use Burns and Kaufman's (1972) interpretation method. This fact makes the comparison of the studies difficult. Some researchers have included variables not previously considered in the original KFD manual. When possible, this author will attempt to distinguish between scoring systems and variables considered.

McGregor (1978) completed one of the most thorough validity studies of the KFD. Using three treatment groups, 157 children, ranging in age from 5 to 13 years, were administered the KFD. Group I was rated as "normal" children by their teacher. Group II consisted of a group of children experiencing conduct problems such as acting-out, aggression, and unmanageable behavior. Group III included children who experienced problems with shyness, phobias, and overly controlling behaviors. Figure omissions were unrelated to a child's age, sex, and problems. McGregor (1978) did not find a relationship between figure size and age, sex, or problems experienced. On the other hand, older children separated their figures significantly more than younger children. Also, "normal" children drew their parents farther apart than either problem group. As compared to Group III, conduct disordered children were more likely to place a barrier between self and father. McGregor (1978) concluded that the KFD was not a valid instrument when discriminating between "normal" and clinically labeled children. Instead of using the KFD for diagnosis, McGregor (1978) recommended that it be used to address behavioral issues that may be significant for the child. Knoff and Prout (1985) noted that McGregor's study had several limitations: (1) validation of the clinical groups' label; (2) neglecting to look at intelligence level and socioeconomic status; and (3) using only two age groupings, even though they have a range of eight years.

McPhee and Wegner (1976) found that the KFD was not a valid instrument when trying to distinguish between normal children and poorly adjusted children. Monahan (1986) supported their findings in that more psychopathology was found in drawings of high achieving children as compared to low achieving children. Additionally, Monahan (1986) noted that the children participating in the success condition (high achieving) spent 40 percent more time completing the KFD. This supported McPhee and Wegner's (1976) finding that well adjusted children spend more time drawing; therefore, they provided more details that fell into Burns and Kaufman's (1972) categories. When comparing a group of children, ranging in age from 6 to 12 years, with behavioral, learning, and emotional problems with a matched group of "normal children", Layton (1983) found no significant differences in the KFD. As with the previous researchers, signs of pathology were found more frequently in the "normal" group.

On the other hand, Sobel and Sobel (1976) discovered that delinquent male adolescents omitted family members more often than "normal" adolescent males. They found that most of the Burns and Kaufman (1972) scoring criteria did not distinguish between the two groups. Rhine (1977) observed that poorly adjusted children showed twice as much compartmentalization and encapsulation as well adjusted children. Again, their results failed to support Burns and Kaufman's (1972) hypotheses of using the KFD to determine adjustment.

Brewer (1980) found significant differences between shy, average, and active children. For instance, shy children drew themselves as isolated whereas active children drew themselves with others (although not interacting). Developmentally delayed children also demonstrated significantly more isolation and rejection when compared to well adjusted children (Raskin & Pitcher-Baker, 1975, 1977; Raskin & Bloom, 1979).

RESEARCH USING THE KFD:

Cabacungan (1985) examined cultural variables related to the KFD. Using a sample of 197 children, 113 Japanese and 84 Filipinos, ranging in age from 9 to 12 years, participated in the study. After the KFDs were administered, names were erased and the drawings were randomly numbered. One Japanese and one Filipino rater used an objective scoring system (Burns, 1982; Thompson, 1975) to rate all 197 drawings. Japanese children significantly drew their actual family size more often than Filipino children. Also, they omitted less characters and added nonmajor figures. Filipino children omitted father and mother figures significantly more often. Both groups drew the mother as the largest figure. Japanese children drew their figures engaging in recreational activities, whereas Filipino children showed figures engaged in work and pleasure. Actions of figures did not reveal cultural or gender differences. Japanese parents were drawn as less communicative as compared to the Filipino children's drawings. Cabacungan (1985) concluded that culture had a significant effect on the drawing of actual family size, actions depicted by major figures, and communication levels of the figures.

Rabinowitz (1991) examined the relationship of acceptance-rejection and KFDs. Although he proposed that peer accepted children would draw themselves closer to other figures than rejected children, the differences were not significant. He did find sex differences in that peer accepted girls drew themselves closer to other figures as compared to boys. The following year, Rabinowitz (1992) examined the height of parental figures in relation to peer acceptance or rejection. The researcher examined 55 boys and 61 girls in the fifth grade. They were given "a sociometric measure consisting of two questions requesting the names of four children with whom the child wished or did not wish to be paired on an outing, and rating of acceptance and rejection were obtained" (Rabinowitz, 1992, p. 329). Rejected children had higher rejection scores than acceptance scores whereas accepted children had higher acceptance scores. Unfortunately, this was the only information given regarding the test used. The nature of this instrument and the subsequent classification of the children was not clear. The researcher then administered the KFD. Sex differences were found only when dividing the children into peer accepted and peer rejected groups: Peer accepted girls drew taller mother and father figures than boys. Rabinowitz (1992) suggested that the family has greater significance for accepted girls than it did for accepted boys. No significant differences were found between peer accepted and rejected boys with respect to the size of parental figures. Accepted girls drew significantly taller mothers than rejected girls. No differences were found with the father figure. Rabinowitz

(1992) concluded that it was important to note peer acceptance/rejection when evaluating the size of parental figures in the KFD.

Stawar and Stawar (1987) researched the possibility of using the KFD as a screening device. They compared the KFD of two groups of white boys who ranged in age from 7 to 11 years. Group I consisted of 18 boys referred to a mental health center for a myriad of issues: learning problems, anxiety, phobias, attention deficit disorder, hyperactivity, and conduct disorders. The children had a full scale IQ above 75. Group II consisted of nine boys enrolled in a public school system who did not suffer from learning, emotional, or behavioral problems. No statistical differences were found between the distance of self to father. Group I boys drew themselves significantly closer to their mothers than Group II boys. The authors also found significant differences in the styles and self actions. For instance, Group I used more edging and encapsulation which is generally associated with isolation, avoidance, and withdrawal. Group II showed more figure underlining and compartmentalization which may suggest feelings of instability and separateness. Group I depicted themselves riding bikes or horses, whereas Group II showed more play. "Although the present results do not support a wholesale endorsement of the test authors' interpretations, they suggest that certain variables (closeness to mother, style, and self-actions) may have potential as components of a screening instrument" (Stawar & Stawar, 1987, p. 810).

Lyons (1993) discussed the use of the KFD in evaluating children in custody cases. When the custody of a child was disputed, Lyons (1993) served as a consultant to provide information on the determination. Her evaluation consisted of four tasks, the second of which will be considered. She used the KFD as a tool since it "appears to be quite directly related to the issues involved in much child forensic work" (Lyons, 1993, p. 156). She examined how the figures were drawn, interaction and space between figures, environmental characteristics, and omissions. When children included a parental figure, it suggested attachment and "may reveal the real and honest need for this family member to remain a part of their emotional life and remain "in the picture'" (Lyons, 1993, p. 158).

Michael and Dudek (1991) examined creativity and mother-child relationships. The researchers assessed the degree of differentiation in both creative and uncreative children using a series of tests. Only the KFD will be considered. Differentiation referred to the mother's ability to encourage the child to develop a separate identity. The initial sample included 133 eight-year-old public school children (60 girls and 73 boys). Using the Torrance Tests of Creative Thinking (TTCT; Torrance, 1966), 15 of the highest scoring children and 15 of the lowest scoring children were selected. Comparing the mothers' interview with the children's KFDs, the researchers found that highly creative children were significantly more differentiated than less creative children.

Much of the research on KFD considered its application to the study of child abuse. Schornstein and Derr (1978) viewed the KFD as a rapid and objective means for determining cases of child abuse and neglect. Their article delineated what they look for in KFDs. For instance, they noted transparencies, stick figures, omissions, and tensions.

> We have also seen the child drawn as a competitor. For example, fathers who draw their sons as being more masculine, aggressive, or larger than themselves, or as being with mother. Child abuse can develop in these instances when the parent regards the child as receiving more attention than the spouse—or an extension of the spouse. (Schornstein & Derr, 1978, p. 35)

Generally, the authors found the KFD was valuable in preventing further abuse and provided information for intervention.

Goodwin (1982) used the KFD when evaluating possible sexual abuse survivors. Although she implemented a series of drawings in the evaluation, only the KFD will be discussed. She examined 19 female children who were suspected sexual abuse survivors. Goodwin (1982) found evidence of isolation, compartmentalization, and role reversals in the drawings of sexual abuse survivors. Additionally, she observed that these children drew themselves larger than their mother.

Hackbarth (1991) et al. found that the KFD can significantly differentiate between abused and nonabused children. Thirty children, ranging in age from 6 to 13 years (mean age of 8.6), classified as sexually abused by the Department of Human Services were compared to 30 unidentified children in a public school district. They ranged in age from 6 to 11 years (mean age of 8.6). The subjects were matched with those in the experimental group: 25 girls and 5 boys (26 were white and 4 were black). Mothers also completed the KFD. Using a Like to Live in Family (LLIF) rating procedure (Burns, 1982), five counselors scored the KFDs on desirability of family life. Sexually abused children drew significantly less desirable family situations compared to their mothers. Mothers of sexually abused children drew significantly less desirable family settings than did mothers of unidentified children. Mothers and their unidentified children did not significantly differ in their KFDs. "The KFD shows enough promise as an evaluation tool in the area of sexual abuse that elementary counselors may want to consider this instrument for inclusion in their repertoire of assessment skills" (Hackbarth et al., 1991, p. 260).

The KFD has revealed common themes in the artwork of sexual abuse survivors. For instance, red houses were typically drawn by sexual abuse survivors (Cohen & Phelps, 1985). Also, children who were sexually abused tend to omit bedrooms or if bedrooms were present, indicated bizarre sleeping arrangements or lack of privacy (Goodwin, 1982). Goodwin (1982) found evidence of isolation, role reversals, and encapsulation in the KFD of sexual abuse survivors. Cohen and Phelps (1985) discovered that the child will often omit self from the KFD. Burgess and Hartman (1993) observed family conflict in KFDs. Isolation, barriers, encapsulation, and sexual themes were also some indicators portrayed in the KFD (German, 1986).

DESIRABLE FEATURES:

The KFD was an interesting approach to understanding the client's perception of self and familial relationships. The grid was a wonderful method of quantifying information about the KFD; yet, the authors did not present guidelines for the interpretation of measurements. The case examples were helpful in understanding how the authors intended the KFD to be used. Overall, the KFD potentially yields valuable information about familial relationships as well as self-concept.

UNDESIRABLE FEATURES:

There was overlap between some of the features of the test. For instance, "light" was used as both a symbol and an action. However, the terms were not clearly defined. Moreover, there was not enough information on how the test was developed, especially the theoretical background. No information was given on who was able to administer the KFD and their qualifications. Interpretation can be difficult given the ambiguity in the test terms and lack of examples for the grid information.

OVERALL EVALUATION:

Although not presented in the manual, objective scoring systems have been developed for the KFD. With training, interrater reliability has been established. However, test-retest reliability evidence was weak suggesting that the KFD may be sensitive to mood changes. Additionally, it may not be a reliable indicator of personality traits.

Validity evidence was also mixed. Research suggested that the KFD cannot distinguish between emotionally disturbed children and well adjusted children. In addition, cultural differences as well as sex differences were found when using the KFD. It was difficult at times to compare validity studies since researchers used a variety of scoring methods. Studies that examined only one variable, such as underling at the bottom, were not considered in this review. Examining only one variable did not seem to provide evidence of an assessment's validity. The exact nature of what the KFD measured was not clear.

The completed summary sheet at the end of the manual can be a useful tool. It would have been more helpful to the reader to have a blank summary sheet. Additionally, the use of the grid to measure size of the figures and distances was helpful. More information was needed on the interpretation of these measurements. Overall, the authors were not clear when outlining the test dimensions. At times, the meanings were ambiguous, such as the distinction between encapsulation and compartmentalization.

The KFD showed promise as a tool that yields information about a child's personality state. It seemed to be a particularly useful tool when evaluating children who were suspected sexual abuse survivors. Further evidence was needed to determine whether or not the KFD can adequately distinguish between other groups such as clinically labeled versus well adjusted children. Overall, the KFD may be a useful approach to gather information about a child's view of self in relationship to family members.

[handwritten margin notes: interpersonal relations; family relations; sexual abuse]

REFERENCES

Brewer, F. (1980). *Children's interaction patterns in Kinetic Family Drawings.* Unpublished doctoral dissertation, United States International University. Cited in Handler & Habenicht (1994).

Burgess, A.W., and Hartman, C.R. (1993). Children's drawings. *Child Abuse & Neglect, 17,* 161–168.

Burns, R.C. (1982). *Self-growth in families.* New York: Brunner/Mazel.

Burns, R.C., and Kaufman, S.H. (1970). *Kinetic Family Drawings (K–F–D): An introduction to understanding children through kinetic drawings.* New York: Brunner/ Mazel.

Burns, R.C., and Kaufman, S.H. (1972). *Actions, styles, and symbols in Kinetic Family Drawings (K–F–D): An interpretive manual.* New York: Brunner/Mazel.

Cabacungan, L.F. (1985). The child's representation of his family in Kinetic Family Drawings (KFD): A cross-cultural comparison. *Psychologia, 28,* 228–236.

Cohen, F.W. and Phelps, R.E. (1985). Incest markers in children's art work. *Arts in Psychotherapy, 12,* 265–284.

Cummings, J.A. (1980). An evaluation of an objective scoring system for the KFDs. *Dissertation Abstracts, 41(6-A),* 2313.

Elin, N., and Nucho, A.O. (1979). The use of kinetic family drawing as a diagnostic tool in assessing the child's self-concept. *Arts in Psychotherapy, 6,* 241–247.

German, D. (1986). *The female adolescent incest victim: Personality, self-esteem, and family orientation.* Unpublished doctoral dissertation, Andrews University. Cited in Handler & Habenicht, 1994.

Goodwin, J. (1982). Use of drawings in evaluating children who may be incest victims. *Children and Youth Services Review, 4,* 269–278.

Hackbarth, S.G., Murphy, H.D., and McQuary, J.P. (1991). Identifying sexually abused children by using Kinetic Family Drawings. *Elementary School Guidance & Counseling, 25,* 225–260.

Handler, L., and Habenicht, D. (1994). The Kinetic Family Drawing technique: A review of the literature. *Journal of Personality Assessment, 62(3),* 440–464.

Knoff, H.M., and Prout, H.T. (1985). The Kinetic Drawing System: A review and integration of the Kinetic Family and School Drawing Techniques. *Psychology in the Schools, 22,* 50–59.

Koppitz, E.M. (1968). *Psychological evaluation of children's human figure drawings.* New York: Grune & Stratton.

Layton, M. (1983). *Special features in the Kinetic Family Drawings of children.* Unpublished doctoral dissertation, Temple University. Cited in Handler & Habenicht, 1994.

Lyons, S.J. (1993). Art psychotherapy evaluations of children in custody disputes. *The Arts in Psychotherapy, 20,* 153–159.

Mangold, J. (1982). *A study of expressions of the primary process in children's Kinetic Family Drawings as a function of pre-drawing activity.* Unpublished doctoral dissertation, Indiana State University. Cited in Handler & Habenicht (1994).

McGregor, J. (1978). *Kinetic Family Drawing Test: A validity study.* Unpublished doctoral dissertation. Auburn University. Cited in Handler & Habenicht (1994).

McPhee, J., and Wegner, K. (1976). Kinetic-Family-Drawing styles and emotionally disturbed childhood behavior. *Journal of Personality Assessment, 40,* 487–491.

Michael, M., and Dudek, S.Z. (1991). Mother-child relationships and creativity. *Creativity Research Journal, 4(3),* 281–286.

Monahan, M. (1986). Situation influences on children's Kinetic Family Drawings. *Dissertation Abstracts International, 46,* 4444.

Mostkoff, D.L., and Lazarus, P.J. (1983). The Kinetic Family Drawing: The reliability of an objective scoring system. *Psychology in the Schools, 20,* 16–20.

Murphy, H.D., and McQuary, J.P. (1991). Identifying sexually abused children by using Kinetic Family Drawings. *Elementary School Guidance & Counseling, 25,* 225–260.

Rabinowitz, A. (1991). The relation of acceptance-rejection to social schemata and Kinetic Family Drawings. *Social Behavior and Personality, 19(4),* 263–272.

Rabinowitz, A. (1992). Acceptance-rejection and height of parental figures on the Kinetic Family Drawings. *Perceptual and Motor Skills, 74,* 329–330.

Raskin, L., and Bloom, A. (1979). Kinetic Family Drawings by children with learning disabilities. *Journal of Pediatric Psychology, 4,* 247–251.

Raskin, L., and Pitcher-Baker, G. (1975). The use of Kinetic Family Drawings in the assessment of children with perceptual-motor delays and developmental disabilities. *Journal of Pediatric Psychology, 3,* 4–5.

Raskin, L., and Pitcher-Baker, G. (1977). Kinetic Family Drawings by children with perceptual-motor delays. *Journal of Learning Disabilities, 10,* 370–374.

Rhine, P. (1977). *Adjustment indicators in Kinetic Family Drawings by children: A validation study.* Unpublished doctoral dissertation, Purdue University. Cited in Handler & Habenicht, 1994.

Schornstein, H.M. and Derr, J. (1978). The many applications of kinetic family drawings in child abuse. *British Journal of Projective Psychology and Personality Study, 23,* 33–35.

Sobel, H., and Sobel, W. (1976). Discriminating adolescent male delinquent through the use of Kinetic Family Drawings. *Journal of Personality Assessment, 40,* 91–94.

Stawar, T.L., and Stawar, D.E. (1987). Family Kinetic Drawings as a screening instrument. *Perceptual and Motor Skills, 65,* 810.

Thompson, L.V. (1975). Kinetic Family Drawings of adolescents. *Dissertation Abstract International, 36(06B),* 3077.

Torrance, E.P. (1966). *Torrance Tests of Creative Thinking: Norms and technical manual.* Princeton, NJ: Personnel Press.

Chapter 4

KINETIC SCHOOL DRAWING

TITLE: Kinetic Drawing System

AGE: age limit for the Kinetic Family Drawing (KFD) is 5 to 20 years whereas the Kinetic School Drawing (KSD) was limited to school aged children

YEAR: 1985

PURPOSE: designed to understand a child's relationships within the family and school setting

SCORES: scoring was based on qualitative interpretations (actions between figures, figure characteristics, distance between figures, drawing style, and symbols)

MANUAL: manual (65 pages); illustrations (18 pages); profile (2 pages); reliability data (1 page); validity data (1 page)

TIME LIMIT: no time limit for administration

COST: $35.00 for testing manual

AUTHOR: Knoff, Howard M., and Prout, H. Thomas

PUBLISHER: Western Psychological Services, 12031 Wilshire Boulevard, Los Angeles, CA, 90025-1251.

INTRODUCTION:

The Kinetic Drawing System (1985) incorporated the Kinetic Family Drawing (KFD; Burns, 1970, 1972). Since the KFD was previously reviewed within this text, only information relating to the Kinetic School Drawing (KSD) will be evaluated. The KSD was designed to investigate the child's psychological status and relationship dynamics within the school setting. The KSD was constructed to reveal a child's attitude toward school.

PURPOSE AND RECOMMENDED USE:

The Kinetic Drawing System (1985) as a whole was used to assess any difficulties that the child was experiencing at home or in school. The system was created to isolate particular relationships that may be contributing to the child's difficulties. Additionally, it was used to identify family issues that may be affecting school behaviors or visa versa. Overall, Knoff and Prout (1985) expressed that the Kinetic Drawing System can serve as a projective technique which investigates the child's personality and perceptions of significant relationships. The authors also stipulated that the system can be used to monitor the child's progress in the counseling setting.

DIMENSIONS THAT THE TEST PURPORTS TO MEASURE:

The dimensions that the KFD measured were discussed previously. The KSD purported to reveal the child's relationships with the instructor and peers. Generally, this section of the test measured the child's attitude toward school. In essence, the KSD manifested the child's concept of self and other self-perceptions as they related to the school milieu.

ADMINISTRATION:

Depending on the individual client, the Kinetic Drawing System may take between 20 and 40 minutes to administer. The authors recommended giving the KFD first and then the KSD, since family issues may affect the child at home and in school. For instance, "a child's self-concept is often primarily determined by his or her interactions with parents (and siblings), their attitudes toward his or her achievement and potential, and the identification process which occurs during the child's early years before school age" (Knoff & Prout, 1985, p. 3). Furthermore, the authors felt that administering the KSD may taint the directions as well as the drawing styles of the KFD. Both the KFD and the KSD consist of a performance phase and an inquiry phase.

The performance phase of the KSD immediately followed the KFD inquiry phase. Here, the child was given the following directions:

> I'd like you to draw a school picture. Put yourself, your teacher, and a friend or two in the picture. Make everyone doing something. Try to draw whole people and make the best drawing you can. Remember, draw yourself, your teacher, and a friend or two, and make everyone doing something. (Knoff & Prout, 1985, p. 4)

In a personal communication to the authors, Burns, one of the creators of the KFD, suggested that the directions read as follows:

> I'd like you to draw a school picture. Put yourself, your teacher, and two or more students in the picture. Try to draw whole people, not stick or cartoon figures. Remember, draw yourself, your teacher, and two or more students doing something. (Knoff & Prout, 1985, p. 4)

Although some children may not feel that they have friends, Knoff and Prout (1985) emphasized that it was important to include the word in the directions since it may reveal clinical information about peer relationships. They also retained the phrase, "make the best drawing you can" because it required a performance demand, similar to the school setting.

The inquiry phase attempted to clarify the child's perception of the drawing. The authors required that the examiner ask the child to describe what was happening in the picture, what each figure was doing, and identify each human or animal figure with a name and age. Although no rigid procedures were required beyond this inquiry, the authors did provide a list of questions that may be helpful in yielding clinical information. The authors did not discuss the qualifications of the examiners. In addition, they did not state if group administration was appropriate.

NORM GROUPS:

Prout and Celmer (1984) examined 100 fifth grade students (44 boys and 56 girls) in a regular education program. It did not appear to be a random sample. Other demographic characteristics of the students were not discussed. The researchers only reported the mean height and distance between figures. For instance, the average height of the teacher was 54.25 mm. The average distance between the self and teacher was 90.00 mm. Although these measurements were interesting, it only revealed information about average fifth grade students. Since the sample was not random, the information may not generalize to other fifth graders. Also, the measurements may not be helpful when evaluating a child older or younger than this sample.

The authors did include normative information from Sarbaugh's (1982) technique for assessing the child's attitude toward school. Although it was not the exact same test, the authors implied that since this assessment was similar to their own, the normative information would be useful. Sarbaugh (1982) examined school aged children, from kindergarten through high school. Knoff and Prout (1985) summarized her work in their manual. For example, Sarbaugh (1982) found that kindergarten students had difficulty with visual-motor coordination. This may be a confounding variable. They also had difficulty putting all of their class members in to the picture. By first grade, children included desks and other features of the classroom. Second grade students featured buildings, rooms, and objects whereas people were de-emphasized. In third grade, students made use of props and equipment. By fourth grade, children drew complete pictures and used more linear perspective. Fifth graders displayed more detail, differentiation of figures, and activities. With junior, middle, and high school students, stick figures were common. Also, drawings were completed more rapidly. This was the extent of the normative information for the KSD.

INTERPRETATION OF SCORES:

Interpretation of the KSD included five diagnostic areas: (1) Actions of and between figures; (2) figure characteristics; (3) position, distance, and barriers; (4) style, and (5) symbols. The qualitative interpretation of the KSD was based on the work of Sarbaugh (1982) and Prout and Celmer (1984). Although Knoff and Prout (1985) warned that the examiner should be sensitive when interpreting the work of special populations, they did not provide guidelines. They stated that drawings completed by learning-disabled, gifted, and behaviorally disturbed children will different from typical children. The nature of these differences and instructions for interpretation for special populations were not discussed.

As for actions of and between figures, the examiner was instructed to look for the self figure engaged in academic behavior. Greater incidence of academic activity was related to greater achievement (Prout & Celmer, 1984). When the self was engaged in disruptive behaviors such as yelling or running, it was associated with lower academic achievement. When a child drew the self in recess activities or nonacademic activities (lunch, music, gym), it may indicate avoidance or anxiety issues.

Figure characteristics were based on the interpretation of subjects drawn in the KFD. Globally, using more than two peers in a drawing was significantly related to lesser academic achievement (Prout and

Celmer, 1984). Lack of people drawn or drawing people symbolically was related to avoidance of social interaction (Sarbaugh, 1982). Large self (greater than 49.25 mm) was significantly related to academic achievement (Prout & Celmer, 1985). If the teacher was larger than self it may reveal feelings of inadequacy. Yet, the authors went on to say that if the teacher was large (greater than 55 mm) it was significantly related to positive academic achievement. This information was contradictory. Excessive detail of the teacher figure was related to possible conflicts, perceptions of a dominating teacher, or authority issues.

Position, distance, and barrier interpretations were based on the KFD (Burns, 1970, 1972). The drawing style of the KSD involved transparencies that may reflect compulsive preoccupations, impulsivity, or poor reality testing. Emphasis of the physical features of a room was said to indicate a need for structure and avoidance of social interaction. Bear in mind that the authors previously stated that second grade students characteristically emphasized the physical features of the room. Children who drew outdoor pictures were said to dislike school and resisted task demands.

The last section focused on a few symbols used in the KSD. For instance, apples may represent oral or dependency needs. Also, apples may symbolize school and teacher activities indicating issues of nurturance and authority. Drawing a school bus was said to indicate avoidance, dislike and conflict of school activities. Also, the authors stated that it served to isolate the child from others. "For a clear analysis, one needs to ask or determine whether the bus is coming to or leaving school and the child's affective relation to either possibility" (Knoff and Prout, 1985, p. 20). Drawing the chalkboard or bulletin board may indicate anxiety about self-adequacy in school. Drawing the principal may reveal conflict with authority or a need for male identification. It was not clear if the authors were assuming that all principals were males.

SOURCE OF ITEMS:

The KSD appeared to be based on the KFD (Burns, 1970, 1972). Interpretation was similar to the KFD. Also, the KSD was related to the work of Sarbaugh (1982) who used a kinetic drawing of the school. It was not clear what similarities and differences existed between Sarbaugh's (1982) school drawing and the KSD.

VALIDITY AND RELIABILITY
AS DETERMINED BY THE AUTHOR:

Reliability of the KSD was not examined by the authors. Validity information was primarily based on the work of other researchers. One study compared Hispanic children with Anglo children who were referred for psychological evaluation. The number of subjects and the manner of selection were not discussed. Using seven objectively scored KSD characteristics, no significant differences were found. The authors concluded that this research indicated that:

> The KSD may be relatively culturally unbiased technique with Hispanics for whom emotional disturbance placement decisions are being considered. At worst, it appears that some KSD style and content characteristics have equal probabilities of occurring on Hispanic or Anglo children's drawings. (Knoff and Prout, 1985, p. 61)

A follow-up study was briefly discussed that examined special populations such as learning disabled and emotionally disturbed children. Since the categorization of the sample was unclear and the methodology limited, Knoff and Prout (1985) did not discuss the implications of the research.

Prout and Celmer (1984) used the KSD to predict academic achievement with 100 fifth grade students. This study was part of the normative information previously discussed. Out of ten KSD variables, six correlated significantly with academic achievement (SRA scores). A large number of peers, overall score, and drawing of self engaged in undesirable behaviors negatively correlated with the SRA scores. Positive correlations involved the child's height, teacher's height, and drawing self engaged in academic behaviors.

The authors included the work of Schneider (1978) who examined the validity of the KSD. Children referred to the school psychologist were assessed. The total sample size and demographic characteristics were not discussed. Schneider (1978) used ratings of the severity of the child's school problems and the severity of the family's problems as dependent measures. Since the KSD could not predict age and IQ, he concluded that his work offered little support of the validity of the KSD.

RESEARCH USING THE KSD:

Andrews and Janzen (1988) developed a scoring sheet and reference guide for the KSD. The scoring sheet was a checklist of 17 items related to the KSD. The reference guide demarcated a list of characteristics that would indicate pathology such as disorganization, distorted body image, and drawing rain to mention a few. Activities were rated as positive, negative, neutral, or uncertain. Guidelines for scoring were discussed. Andrews and Janzen (1988) also constructed a rating scale to determine the degree of behavioral issues such as depression, aggression, isolation, etc. They examined an equal number of learning disabled (LD) and non learning disabled (NLD) children in fifth grade attending eight different schools. A total of 96 drawings were examined by two sets of three trained raters. Interrater reliability was reported to be above .70. Significantly more NLD children showed structure in their drawings. Significantly more LD drawings indicated negative interactions with peers and instructors. Also, they depicted themselves more often outside of school and involved in nonacademic activities or undesirable forms of behavior compared to NLD students. Significantly more LD children were rated as depressed, impulsive, and competitive. The scoring sheet, reference guide, and rating scale were able to differentiate between the two groups of students. The authors concluded that their instruments demonstrated reliability and some discriminant validity.

Neale and Rosal (1993) evaluated a series of projective assessments. In reviewing the literature, some of which was previously discussed, Neale and Rosal (1993) found that the KSD indicated strong concurrent validity when correlated with achievement measures. The authors evaluated the research based on problem, design, procedure, and analysis. Based on the research on KSD validity, the authors gave the instrument 46 points out of a possible 50 points.

DESIRABLE FEATURES:

The KSD was easy to administer and did not require much time. The manual included several case examples which were helpful when interpreting drawings. Overall, the manual was easy to read and clear.

UNDESIRABLE FEATURES:

Interpretation of the KSD may be difficult. Only qualitative information was considered. A scoring guide that was objective in nature would have been more helpful. At times, the information appeared contradictory. For instance, the authors stated that drawing a large teacher was related to feelings of inadequacy in school. In the next paragraph, they stated that drawing a large teacher was related to positive school achievement. How can one adequately interpret school achievement based on the size of the instructor given this information? Normative information was lacking. Also, guidelines for interpreting the drawings completed by special populations was non existent.

OVERALL EVALUATION:

The reliability of the KSD was not established in the manual. Andrews and Janzen (1988) did create a scoring guide, reference sheet, and rating scale that demonstrated some reliability. Additional information regarding the stability of the KSD was needed.

Overall, the KSD did demonstrate some concurrent validity. Discriminant validity information was needed. For example, it would be helpful to know how emotionally disturbed children's KSDs differ from children who were not diagnosed with emotional disorders. Guidelines for the interpretation of drawings from special populations should be established.

The normative information was weak. Although there was a normative study of fifth grade students, norms were not established for other age groups. Since the normative sample was unreliable, the interpretation of the KSD was difficult. Additionally, the authors used a norm sample from a test that was similar to their own. It cannot be assumed that these assessments were similar. Additionally, it cannot be assumed that the normative information from Sarbaugh's (1982) work will be useful when interpreting the KSD.

As opposed to Neale and Rosal's (1993) findings, I did not agree that the KSD was a valid instrument. Although the manual did report some concurrent validity, additional research was required. There was not enough information on the KSD to warrant its use within the school or counseling settings.

REFERENCES

Andrews, J., and Janzen, H. (1988). A global approach for the interpretation of the Kinetic School Drawing (KSD): A quick scoring sheet, reference guide, and rating scale. *Psychology in the schools, 25,* 217-237.

Burns, R.C., and Kaufman, S.H. (1970). *Kinetic Family Drawings (K–F–D): An introduction to understanding children through kinetic drawings.* New York: Brunner/Mazel.

Burns, R.C., and Kaufman, S.H. (1972). *Actions, styles, and symbols in Kinetic Family Drawings (K–F–D): An interpretive manual.* New York: Brunner/Mazel.

Knoff, H.M., and Prout, H.T. (1985). *Kinetic Drawing System for Family and School: A handbook.* Los Angeles, CA: Western Psychological Services.

Knoff, H.M., and Prout, H.T. (1985). The Kinetic Drawing System: A review and integration of the kinetic family and school drawing techniques. *Psychology in the Schools, 22,* 50-59.

Neale, E.L., and Rosal, M.L. (1993). What can art therapists learn from the research on projective drawing techniques for children? A review of the literature. *The Arts in Psychotherapy, 20,* 37-49.

Prout, H.T., and Celmer, D.S. (1984). School drawings and academic achievement: A validity study of the Kinetic School Drawing technique. *Psychology in the Schools, 21,* 176-180.

Sarbaugh, M.E.A. (1982). Kinetic Drawing-School (KD-S) Technique. *Illinois School Psychologists' Association Monograph Series, 1,* 1-70.

Schneider, G.B. (1978). A preliminary validation study of the Kinetic School Drawing. *Dissertation Abstracts International, 38,* 6628A.

Chapter 5

DIAGNOSTIC DRAWING SERIES

TITLE:	Diagnostic Drawing Series (DDS)
AGE:	adolescents and adults
YEAR:	1986
PURPOSE:	designed to link picture analysis to DSM–III and DSM--III–R diagnoses: Assesses an individual's response to structured and unstructured drawing tasks
SCORES:	interpretation was based on a rating guide (considers 23 variables for rating)
MANUAL:	rating guide (10 pages); reliability data (none reported); validity data (none reported)
TIME LIMIT:	15-minute time limit for each drawing task for a total of 45 minutes
COST:	$2.00 for handbook; $2.00 for rating guide
AUTHOR:	Cohen, Barry M.
PUBLISHER:	Cohen, Barry M., PO Box 9853, Alexandria, VA, 22304.

INTRODUCTION:

The Diagnostic Drawing Series (DDS) was designed to gather clinical information about a client in a single session. By presenting structured and unstructured drawing tasks, the DDS provided information toward the clarification of DSM–III and DSM–III–R diagnoses. "This instrument was created because of the clinical imprecision of existing art therapy assessment procedures and the absence of a research foundation on which to base clinical judgments" (Mills et al., 1993, p. 83). The DDS can be used by art therapists and mental health professionals alike. Additionally, it was compatible with psychiatric diagnostic research.

PURPOSE AND RECOMMENDED USE:

The DDS was designed to be used in clinical settings. When assessing adolescents and adults, the DDS reflected behavioral and affective states of the client. Also, the DDS provided information about the client's strengths, defenses, and issues. Within three to five days of admission to a mental health center, the DDS was administered to the client. Cohen (1985) recommended that two psychiatrists or one psychiatrist and one psychologist fill out a psychiatric diagnosis form to be used in conjunction with the DDS. The information obtained from the three drawing tasks was correlated with the DSM diagnoses. The DDS can be used in individual sessions, group therapy, educational planning, and as a guide in treatment and termination (Cohen, Mills, Kijak, 1994). A 15-minute time limit for each drawing as well as strict adherence to administration requirements were recommended.

DIMENSIONS THAT THE TEST PURPORTS TO MEASURE:

The initial, free drawing purported to measure the defensive functioning of the client. Additionally, the free drawing indicated the individual's response to an unstructured task. The second directive, the tree drawing, "provides a rich portrait of the individual's vegetative/psychic state" (Cohen, 1985, p. 2). This structured task yielded information about the person's life energy or life force (Burns, 1987). According to Cohen (1985), the tree drawing can be used as a diagnostic aid when considering organic impairment. The last directive, "make a picture of how you are feeling," revealed the client's affective state.

> This semi-structured task allows for self-assertion and self-reflection by the patient. The feeling picture also promotes abstract thinking. (Cohen, 1985, p. 2)

As with the first drawing, this task may gauge flexibility and defensive functioning of the client.

Pictorial characteristics, such as line, color, and shape, were rated and correlated with the client's psychiatric diagnosis. Twenty-three variables were outlined and used to rate each drawing. For instance, when viewing a DDS drawing, the number of colors used, blending, and the use of idiosyncratic colors were noted. Method of representation, integration, and line quality were also recorded. Rather than "measuring" these variables, the author suggested noting their presence or absence.

ADMINISTRATION:

The administration requirements for the DDS were clearly delineated. Within three days (no more than five days) of admission to a psychiatric setting, the patient should complete the DDS. A strict, 15-minute time limit was used for each drawing task. A box of 12 Alphacolor square pastels, three sheets of 18 × 24 inch (60 lb) white drawing paper, and Krylon Crystal Clear spray fixative were required. The person was told, "the page may be turned in any direction. Make a picture using these materials." When the first drawing was complete, the administrator immediately preceded with the second drawing: "Make a picture of a tree." This was completed even if the patient drew a tree in the first picture. The last directive was "Make a picture of how you're feeling, using lines, shapes, and colors." If a patient could not complete a drawing, a blank picture was considered. The patient's verbal associations were recorded following the last drawing task.

NORM GROUPS:

The DDS handbook and rating guide contained little information on the groups used to standardize the assessment. It appeared that the DDS was standardized on a clinical population, in one particular hospital. This information may not generalize to other settings. More information was needed on the population used to develop the DDS. A later article was said to have established norms for the DDS; yet, the demographic characteristics of this sample were not discussed (Cohen, Hammer, and Singer, 1988).

INTERPRETATION OF SCORES:

The DDS drawings were rated using a guide created by Cohen (1986). The Drawing Analysis Form (DAF) may be used to record the information for each drawing in the series. Interpretation of the DDS may be difficult. Other than noting the presence or absence of the variables listed, no other interpretive guidelines were discussed in the rating manual or the handbook. Cohen (1986) clearly delineated the categories for rating the DDS; yet, failed to provide adequate guidelines for the interpretation of these variables.

SOURCE OF ITEMS:

Since Cohen (1985) did not discuss the historical and theoretical development of the DDS, the exact source of the items was unclear. The first exercise, a free drawing, was an activity used by some of the founders of art therapy (Kwiatkowska, 1978; Wadeson, 1980; & Naumburg, 1987). Free pictures were unstructured drawing tasks for which no subject was assigned. Kwiatkowska (1978) stressed that the free drawing contained the most important information about the client. The client's ego strength, defenses, and presenting issues often appeared in free drawings. Cohen (1985) related the first picture to the analysis of a first dream in that "the picture represents what the individual is willing to initially share of himself" (p. 2).

Cohen (1985) stated that the second directive was linked to the projective tree tests of the past:

> The tree is an ancient symbol and has been studied in the context of projective drawings. The tree symbol represents the deepest tapping of the psyche in the realm of projective drawing subject matter. (p. 2)

Assessments that describe personality based on tree drawings have been developed by a number of therapists (Buck, 1948; Bolander, 1977; Burns, 1987). A few of these tests have been reviewed within this text.

The last drawing task appeared to be originally created by the author. It was a semistructured task designed to evoke the affective state of the client. Additional information on the source of this task would be helpful.

VALIDITY AS DETERMINED BY THE AUTHOR:

Reliability and validity information was not discussed in the handbook or the rating guide. In a separate article, 239 patients from the Fairfax Hospital completed the DDS (Cohen, Hammer, & Singer; 1988). The demographic characteristics of the sample were not presented. The researchers did not utilize a random sample. Although the authors stated that only 239 cases were available for the study, it was not clear how these cases were separated into the four groups: schizophrenia, depression, dysthymia, and nonpatients. When the authors presented the tables for each of these groups, they present an N = 239 for each group. Other than the nonpatient group, it was not clear if a case was represented in more than one category. Significant differences in the DDS were discussed for each group. For instance, dysthymia patients used light pressure, included animals in the free drawing, and drew disintegrated trees. Depressed patients showed unusual placement of images on the page, a characteristic not demonstrated by the other groups. In addition, depressed people lacked a landscape in the tree picture and included water images in the feeling picture. Schizophrenic patients drew monotone feeling pictures. Also, they lacked integration in the free picture and depicted short tree trunks. The overall significance level for each group was below .05. This may indicate that the DDS differentiated client populations.

RELIABILITY AS DETERMINED BY THE AUTHOR:

Interrater reliability was determined by examining 30 DDSs. The source of these drawings was unclear. After a two-month training period, Cohen, an experienced art therapist, and Meneses, a nonart therapist, rated each series. Interrater reliability was reported to be 95.7 percent (Mills, Cohen, & Meneses, 1993). The lowest agreement (.77) was with the category of representation. The remainder of the categories indicated agreement in the 1990s. The study would have been more objective had Cohen not included himself as a rater.

RESEARCH USING THE DDS:

In the DDS handbook, Cohen (1985) stated that the DDS was helpful when diagnosing organic dysfunction. He did not provide further information regarding this statement. In 1994, Couch used the DDS when working with elderly people with organic mental syndromes and disorders. Using DSM–III–R criteria, 24 patients (16 females and 8 males) suffering from organic dysfunction were given the DDS. They ranged in age from 63 to 93 years. A control sample of ten subjects with no organic dysfunction completed the DDS. One-half of the subjects were given the DDS in a group setting whereas the other one-half were administered individually. The participants were in the course of treatment at the time the research was conducted. Two art therapists trained to administer the DDS rated all three pictures. The researcher found that the treatment sample tended to use only one color, single images, and light line pressure. Trees were generally unrecognizable. Also, the pictures were impoverished with minimal inclusion of animals or people. Floating images, limited use of space, and unusual placement on the page characterized the organically impaired group. Pictures became more disorganized as the session progressed. Couch (1994) did note the limitations of the study: use of one racial group, raters were not blind to diagnoses, and the lack of a random sample. In conclusion, Couch (1994) stated that the DDS can be helpful when diagnosing possible cases of organic dysfunction.

Knapp (1994) used the DDS when working with Alzheimer patients. Subjects were recruited from an ongoing treatment and research population. Fifty subjects matched by age participated in the study. The Alzheimer patients were early in the course of the illness and evidenced pathology (mean age of 69 with 9 males and 16 females). The control group did not suffer from psychiatric or medical disorders (mean age of 71 with 10 males and 15 females). Although Knapp (1994) used other assessments, only the results of the DDS will be considered. Knapp (1994) created a checklist of 39 variables that was used by three independent art therapists. A total of 195 drawings were scored yielding a 90 percent agreement among raters. "Criterion-related validity was provided by establishing the 39 variables in the Graphic Indicator List from diagnostic criteria from the DSM–III–R for Primary Degenerative Dementia of the Alzheimer Type, since that constellation of symptoms distinguished the AD group of subjects from the control subjects" (Knapp, 1994, p. 134). The Alzheimer patients used fewer colors and less space compared to the control subjects. Knapp (1994) did not make a final conclusion regarding the use of the DDS.

Kessler (1994) used the DDS with a group of eating disordered subjects. People were selected from an inpatient eating disordered program for women. The group included 55 women with Bulimia Nervosa, 17 with Anorexia Nervosa, and nine with Eating Disorder NOS. They were diagnosed in accordance to DSM–III–R criteria. Other demographic characteristics of the sample were not discussed. Drawings were obtained in a group format within five days of admission to the center. Kessler (1994) used the DAF to note the occurrence and nonoccurrence of the DDS criteria. The combined sample showed significantly less use of a groundline. Also, the group drew trees that were falling apart and had knotholes. Kessler (1994) concluded that the DDS might be helpful in establishing a tentative diagnosis for eating disorders.

Neale (1994) developed the Children's Diagnostic Drawing Series (CDDS) with a clinical population. A sample of 100 children from a private school served as the control group. A sample of 80 children from an outpatient mental health center comprised the treatment group. Neale (1994) clearly outlined the demographic characteristics of the sample. Additionally, she described the clinical diagnoses of the treatment group including the number of subjects in each category. These subjects were randomly selected from a larger pool. The CDDS differed from the DDS in that it used hard pastels and modified the instructions slightly. Instead of the original directive, "Make a picture using these materials," the administrator stated, "Make a picture using the pastels and paper." The drawings were collected in group and individual sessions. Using the 23 variables from the rating guide, the author and two trained DDS raters (blind to the study) evaluated the drawings. Twelve variables showed significant interrater reliability. Seven variables distinguished between the control and treatment groups: color type, line/shape, integration, groundline, inanimate objects, abstract symbols, and space usage. The clinical group drawings were impoverished, lacked a groundline, used only one color, and used less space. In addition, the author found that 20 variables significantly described children diagnosed with adjustment disorder. Although Neale (1994) noted the limitations of the study, she did an excellent job of describing the subjects, outlining the method, and summarizing the results.

DESIRABLE FEATURES:

One advantage of using the DDS was that three drawings can be obtained in one session. The DDS employed one medium yet allowed for the examination of color. The combination of structured and unstructured drawing tasks generated information about the client's defenses and response to directives.

UNDESIRABLE FEATURES:

The interpretation of the DDS may be difficult. Other than noting the presence or absence of pictorial characteristics, the handbook and rating guide did not provide information related to diagnostic categories. Another possible limitation was the time factor. The pressure of completing a drawing in 15 minutes may cause stress and anxiety in some people. This has not been examined in the research on the DDS.

OVERALL EVALUATION:

The DDS was a tool that may be helpful in providing clinical information related to diagnosis. Research on the DDS, to date, has shown that it can distinguish between clinical populations and "normal" populations. This was true of the CDDS as well. People with adjustment disorders, depression, dysthymia, schizophrenia, and organic syndromes have drawing styles characteristically different than well adjusted individuals. The DDS also showed promise in providing indications of eating disorders.

Given that Cohen has completed research on the DDS, it would be helpful if he rewrote the handbook in accordance with the Standards for Educational and Psychological Testing (AERA, APA, NCME, 1985). A section on the historical development and the theoretical background of the assessment would be beneficial. Particularly important was information on the sample used to norm the DDS. The author should provide guidelines for the interpretation of the DDS.

Overall, the DDS may be a valuable tool to provide information on clinical diagnoses. A desirable feature was that the assessment can be completed in one session. By changing the rating guide to a Likert scale or continuous scale, statistical analysis for the DDS would be enhanced. With these changes in the rating guide and the handbook, the DDS would surpass other art therapy assessments in standardization, validity, and reliability.

REFERENCES

American Educational Research Association, American Psychological Association, & National Council on Measurement in Education. (1985). *Standards for educational and psychological testing.* Washington, DC: American Psychological Association.

Bolander, K. (1977). *Assessing personality through tree drawings.* New York: Basic Books.

Buck, J.N. (1948). *The House-Tree-Person Technique.* Los Angeles, CA: Western Psychological Services.

Burns, R.C. (1987). *Kinetic-House-Tree-Person-Drawings: An interpretive manual.* New York: Brunner/Mazel.

Cohen, B.M. (Ed.). (1985). *The Diagnostic Drawing Series Handbook.* Alexandria, VA: Barry Cohen.

Cohen, B.M. (Ed.). (1986). *The Diagnostic Drawing Series Rating Guide.* Alexandria, VA: Barry Cohen.

Cohen, B.M., Hammer, J.S., and Singer, S. (1988). The Diagnostic Drawing Series: A systematic approach to art therapy evaluation and research. *The Arts in Psychotherapy, 15,* 11–21.

Cohen, B.M., Mills, S., and Kijak, A.K. (1994). An introduction to the Diagnostic Drawing Series: A standardized tool for the diagnostic and clinical use. *Art Therapy, 11(2)*, 105–110.

Couch, J.B. (1994). Diagnostic Drawing Series: Research with older people diagnosed with organic mental syndromes and disorders. *Art Therapy, 11(2)*, 111–115.

Kessler, K. (1994). A study of the Diagnostic Drawing Series with eating disordered patients. *Art Therapy, 11(2)*, 116–118.

Knapp, N.M. (1994). Research with Diagnostic Drawings for normal and Alzheimer's subjects. *Art Therapy, 11(2)*, 131–138.

Kwiatkowska, H.Y. (1978). *Family therapy and evaluation through art.* Springfield, IL: Charles C Thomas.

Mills, A., Cohen, B.M., and Meneses, J.Z. (1993). Reliability and validity tests of the Diagnostic Drawing Series. *The Arts in Psychotherapy, 20*, 83–88.

Naumburg, M. (1987). *Dynamically oriented art therapy: Its principles and practices.* Chicago, IL: Magnolia Street Publishers.

Neale, E.L. (1994). The Children's Diagnostic Drawing Series. *Art Therapy, 11(2)*, 119–126.

Wadeson, H. (1980). *Art psychotherapy.* New York: John Wiley & Sons.

Chapter 6

HOUSE TREE PERSON TEST

TITLE: House Tree Person Test (HTP)
AGE: age limit not presented
YEAR: 1987
PURPOSE: designed to provide information on personality characteristics and interpersonal relationships
SCORES: scoring was based on the presence or absence of features associated with detail, proportion, and perspective; interpretation was based on drawing characteristics such as color, line, placement on the page, etcetera; two forms of test (chromatic and achromatic); quantitatively and qualitatively scored
MANUAL: manual (350 pages); illustrations (58 pages); profile (6 pages); reliability data (none reported); validity data (none reported)
TIME LIMIT: no time limit for individual administration; 90 time limit for group administration
COST: $58.00–65.00 for testing manual
AUTHOR: Buck, John N.
PUBLISHER: Western Psychological Services., 12031 Wilshire Boulevard, Los Angeles, CA, 90025.

INTRODUCTION:

The House Tree Person Test (HTP) was designed to provide information on the client's personality. According to Buck (1987), the HTP yielded details on the client's "sensitivity, maturity, flexibility, efficiency, degree of personality integration, and interactions with the environment" (p. 1). Also, the HTP represented the client's level of intellectual functioning. In Phase One of the HTP, the client used pencil to create a house, tree, and a person on separate sheets of paper. Phase Two was structured and verbal. The client used crayons to draw a house, tree, and person. This part of the assessment involved client associations to the objects drawn.

PURPOSE AND RECOMMENDED USE:

Generally, the HTP was designed to furnish knowledge on the client's personality, behavior patterns, and interpersonal interactions. "The author feels strongly that the H–T–P may be employed usefully in individual examinations to provide the clinical psychologist, psychiatrist, or other qualified examiner with diagnostically and prognostically significant data concerning Ss [subjects] which otherwise might take much more time to acquire" (Buck, 1987, p. 2). In addition, Buck (1987) stated that the HTP may be used as a measure of change during the course of therapy. He felt that the HTP may be utilized as a screening device to measure maladjustment, appraise personality integration, and identify common personality characteristics of a specific population. Also, he expressed that the HTP can serve as a pretest tool for entrance into a school, specialized training program, or an employment position.

DIMENSIONS THAT THE TEST PURPORTS TO MEASURE:

The HTP measured an individual's response to an ambiguous task. Like other projective techniques, the HTP evoked projective material from the client. It accomplished this in a verbal as well as a nonverbal fashion. Additionally, the HTP calibrated intellectual functioning. Details, proportion, perspective, concept formation, and vocabulary comprised the appraisal of intellectual functioning. Each section of the test (house, tree, and person) was viewed as a psychological self-portrait. Buck (1987) asserted that the HTP stimulates conscious, subconscious, and unconscious associations. Since the house was the place of the client's most intimate interpersonal relationships, this part of the test suggested associations concerning the home and those living in the home. Teillard (1951) believed that the house represented the layers of the psyche: The outside symbolized the person's appearance, the upper floor exemplified conscious control, and the cellar depicted the unconscious. According to Buck (1987), the tree fostered associations concerning the person's life-role and satisfaction with the environment. Essentially, Buck (1949) viewed the tree as a symbol of the psychological development of the person with infancy at the bottom and present life age at the top.

> The roots refer to the relationship to reality, the trunk to ego strength, and the branches and foliage refer to the ability to interact satisfactorily with the environment. A knothole indicates a traumatic event. (Ramirez, 1983, p. 44)

Essentially, the tree portrayed the person's psychological age. This section of the test aroused associations to past, present, and future interpersonal relationships.

> Any emotion exhibited by the S [subject] while drawing or being questioned concerning his drawings is presumed to represent an emotional reaction to the relationships, situations, needs or presses, or other dynamics which the S [subject] feels are directly or symbolically represented or suggested by one or more of his drawings or a part thereof. (Buck, 1987, p. 4)

Color use and affective reaction related to the client's tolerance, control, and response to emotionally arousing stimuli. Comparison of the chromatic and achromatic forms of the test provided information on the constancy of intellectual functioning as well as attitudes, emotional reactions, and other behaviors.

ADMINISTRATION:

Drawings were completed on white paper (6 sheets) 7 by 8 1/2 inches. Several No. 2 lead pencils and a set of wax crayons (including red, green, blue, yellow, brown, black, purple, and orange) were required. A stopwatch and the four page HTP Scoring Folder was also necessary.

The administrator began with the achromatic drawings. For the house drawing, the paper was placed horizontally with the word, HOUSE, written at the top of the page. For the tree and person drawings, the page was placed vertically. The following directive was given:

> Take one of these pencils, please. I want you to draw me as good a picture of a house as you can. You may draw any kind of house you wish, it's entirely up to you. You may erase as much as you like, it will not be counted against you. And you may take as long as you wish, Just draw me as good a house as you can. (Buck, 1987, p. 18)

If the client objected due to his artistic abilities, the administrator explained that the HTP was not a test of artistic talent. Since the drawing must be freehand, the subject was not permitted to use a ruler. After giving the instructions, the administrator started the stopwatch. The initial latency period between the instructions and drawing, name and number of details, pauses, spontaneous comments, affect, and total time used to complete the drawing were recorded. The same procedure was followed for the tree and person drawings.

After the last drawing was complete, the therapist administered the Post-Drawing Interrogation (PDI). This gave the client an opportunity to describe, define, and interpret the objects drawn and give associations concerning them. The interrogation contained 60 questions and were labeled by object (H,T,P). Additional labels included A for Association, P for Pressure, and R for Reality testing. Pressure referred to any factors that may have a positive or negative influence on the client's behavior. For example, question T6 (tree question) read, "which does that Tree look more like to you: a man or a woman? (A & R)" (p. 22). This question apparently evoked associations and assessed reality testing. Buck (1987) stressed that the administrator should not adhere strictly to the PDI since other questions may arise during the assessment.

After the PDI, the chromatic drawings were completed. The administrator presented a set of crayons to the client and asked her to identify the colors. This was done to check for possible color blindness. The administrator followed the procedure used for the achromatic version of the test. After the last drawing was complete, the therapist administered the chromatic PDI as long as the client was not too fatigued after drawing. This interrogation contained 22 questions broken down by test section: House, Tree, and Person.

For group administration, 90 minutes was allotted. The therapist recorded the time used by each person to complete the sections of the test, affect displayed, questions asked, and comments. With the PDI, the group was asked to write their responses down after the questions were asked. Next, the chromatic version of the test was administered. Subjects identified colors by making check marks in the lower left corner of the page. The same procedure for the achromatic section of the test was followed. Administrator qualifications were not discussed.

NORM GROUPS:

Subjects were selected to represent the following intelligence categories: imbecile, moron, borderline, dull average, average, above average, and superior. Twenty subjects represented each category. The people participating in the imbecile through average levels were white residents, patients, or employees of the Lynchburg State Colony. The average group consisted of college students in Nebraska and Virginia. They had completed at least two years of college. Superior subjects were graduate students in a medical program. Buck (1987) presented a table listing the groups' intellectual level, gender, education achievement, and life age.

Using the individual administration guidelines that were previously discussed, 100 sets of drawings were obtained from the less than above average group. Group administration was used for the above average and superior groups. Group administration differed from individual administration in that subjects were presented with a triple problem at once whereas the individual administration focused on only one section of the test at a time. Also, the group administration involved writing comments about the drawings subsequent to the completion of the task.

A total of 140 sets of drawing were analyzed to identity and list items that may distinguish intelligence level. Detail, proportion, and perspective appeared to differentiation the subjects. Buck (1987) then provided definitions of detail, proportion, and perspective. Next the drawings were rated as "good" or "flaw." A "good" item referred to as an item of detail, proportion, and perspective used by 50 percent of the sample and by less than 50 percent of the subjects below the borderline level. A "flaw" item was defined as an item presented by at least 50 percent of the group rated less than borderline intelligence and by less than 50 percent of the subjects from the borderline group and up.

Factor symbols were then assigned to the drawings. The letter D was assigned to those items of detail, proportion, or perspective used by at least 50 percent of the subjects of one of the "flaw" groups and by less than 50 percent of the subjects of each higher group. The letter A was assigned to those items used by at least 50 percent of the people of one of the levels borderline through average and by less than 50 percent of the people in the upper levels. The letter S denoted those items used by 50 percent or more of the above average or superior groups and by less than 50 percent of the people in each lower level groups. For example, Buck (1987) found that 15 percent of the subjects in the imbecile group, 30 percent of the moron group, 30 percent of the borderline group, 60 percent of the dull average group, 65 percent of the average group, and 95 percent of the above average and superior groups drew houses with more than one window.

The next sample involved a qualitative analysis of items that distinguished maladjustment as opposed to intelligence. A total sample of 150 people from two clinical settings completed the HTP. "The S [subject] population . . . indicated definitely that the H–T–P productions of Ss [subjects] with personality disorders differed in many respects from drawings produced by Ss who were not maladjusted" (Buck, 1987, p. 14). The well-adjusted group was not discussed. Detail, proportion, perspective, time, comments, associations, line quality, self-criticisms, attitude, drive, and concept served to differentiate between maladjusted individuals and well adjusted people. How this determination was made was unclear. Additionally, the people involved in making the analysis of the drawings for this study and the previous study, along with their qualifications were not discussed. The breakdown of the subjects into the intellectual levels and the diagnostic categories was not clear.

INTERPRETATION OF SCORES:

The HTP may be scored quantitatively as well as qualitatively. The scoring for each method was clearly described and included illustrated case examples. The quantitative method viewed the detail, proportion, and perspective factors of each section of the test. For the house, tree, and person, the total scores were computed for the following categories: D3, D2, D1, A1, A2, A3, S1, S2. These categories were directly linked to the standardization sample and represented intellectual functioning. For instance, house drawing that lacked a roof was labeled D3 as representative of individuals with inferior intelligence. A house drawing that included roof material (shading, blocking, diagonal lines, etcetera) was labeled as S1, indicating superior intelligence. In addition to the verbal descriptions of the categories, Buck (1987) incorporated illustrations of the various possibilities. Raw scores were weighted to determine good scores and flaw scores. Overall, this method provided an indication of intellectual functioning. Buck (1987) furnished guidelines for interpreting the HTP IQ in relation to other standardized measures of intelligence.

Qualitative analysis considered details (relevant and irrelevant), proportion, and perspective. In addition, time consumption, line quality, criticality, attitude, drive, and color were examined. These sections were thoroughly outlined. For instance, the category of perspective involved placement on the page. When the tree drawing appeared in the upper portion of the paper, it indicated a person who was prone to fantasy, set unattainable goals, and felt frustrated. A tree placed in the lower portion of the page may reveal a person who felt insecure and may be mildly depressed. Guidelines for qualitative analysis were clearly outlined.

SOURCE OF ITEMS:

Buck (1987) stated that the objects of the house, tree, and person were selected because they were familiar items for very young children as well as adults. Additionally, he felt that these objects were more accepted by clients of all ages compared to other suggested objects. Lastly, he found that the house, tree, and person seemed to foster more open and free associations than did other items. The nature of the "other suggested objects" was not discussed.

VALIDITY AND RELIABILITY AS DETERMINED BY THE AUTHOR:

Buck (1987) did not present reliability and validity studies to support the use of the HTP. Several pilot studies have been conducted using the HTP. Unfortunately, these studies did not concentrate on establishing reliability and validity evidence. Nonetheless, they did provide information on the usefulness of this assessment.

RESEARCH USING THE HTP:

Kline and Svaste-Xuto (1981) examined the cultural implications of the HTP. A total sample of 80 Thai children, ranging in age from 4 to 6 years, completed the HTP. A total of 40 British children of the same age completed the HTP. The samples were not random nor matched and therefore, represented a restricted population. Further demographic characteristics of the subjects were not discussed. The drawings were scored for the presence or absence of features. For instance, the following was an example of how the authors scored a drawing of a tree:

BRANCHES:	presence of branches = 1 pt.,	absence = 0
BARK:	presence of bark = 1 pt.,	absence = 0
ROOTS:	presence of roots = 1 pt.,	absence = 0

The authors reported that the scoring system they developed was highly reliable, showing 90 percent agreement. The PDI questions were also objectively scored. Sex differences were found in the Person drawings: Significantly more Thai girls indicated that their person was a young, healthy, woman. The authors expressed that this supported the validity of Buck's statement that children were more likely to draw a person of the same sex. Significantly more girls said that their house had one or two stories. No sex differences were found in tree drawings. Cultural differences were not found. The authors concluded that the HTP, when objectively scored, was a suitable personality assessment for cross-cultural use.

The HTP has been used to investigate physical abuse cases (Lewis & Goldstein, 1981). A sample 109 children completed the HTP. The physically abused-clinical group consisted of 32 children participating in therapy for child abuse (physical). A sample of 32 children, judged by their therapists not to have been physically abused, comprised the nonabused-clinical group. The "normal" group consisted of 45 children from a local elementary school, judged by their teachers to be highly well adjusted and to come from homes where physical abuse was unlikely. The authors found that the following items occurred significantly more often in the abused-clinical group than the other two: smoke coming from the chimney, absence of windows on the ground floor of the house, noticeable difference in the arms and legs of figures, and absence of feet, and disproportional size of the head. In conclusion, the authors stipulated that the items taken individually strongly distinguish between abused and normal children but not between abused and nonabused but disturbed children. This study may provide some validity evidence that the HTP distinguished between well adjusted children and maladjusted children.

Ramirez (1983) examined the usefulness of the HTP in working through resistance in group settings. Resistance was defined as the conscious, preconscious, or unconscious opposition that envelops one's attitudes, ideas, impulses, thoughts, actions, and fantasies (Greenson, 1967). Ramirez (1983) presented case examples of groups where resistance impeded therapeutic progress. "The house, tree, and person drawing task is especially useful for group therapists unfamiliar with art therapy techniques because there is a large body of work available for help in interpreting the images and because patients have been found to be less resistant to drawing these particular subjects, which are familiar to everyone's experience" (Ramirez, 1983, p. 48). Although this study was qualitative in its approach, it illustrated how the HTP may be helpful in overcoming resistance patterns by reducing defensiveness and promoting group discussion.

Marzolf and Kirchner (1972) collected HTPs from 760 college students (454 women and 306 men) enrolled in psychology courses. On the same day or a few weeks later, the students were given the Sixteen

Personality Factor Questionnaire Form C (Catell, 1962). The authors prepared a list of 108 characteristics of HTP drawings. All drawings were analyzed for the presence or absence of these characteristics. Using two assistants, the interrater reliability was better than 90 percent. Thirty-six percent of the 108 items showed sex differences. In relationship to the questionnaire, no reliable differences were found between those judged as disturbed and more well adjusted individuals. Due to the sex differences found in the items, the authors underscored the importance of inquiry when interpreting the drawing.

Ouellette (1988) administered the HTP to 33 young deaf adults. Psychologists rated the drawings on scales measuring, aggression, anxiety, insecurity, impulsiveness, immaturity, egocentricity, dependency, and feelings of inadequacy. Interrater reliability was established for aggression, impulsiveness, immaturity, and feelings of inadequacy. By comparing psychologists' ratings of the drawings with trained counselors' clinical observations, validity was established for five personality trait scales: aggression, impulsiveness, immaturity, egocentricity, and dependency. In conclusion, Ouellette (1988) stressed that "while the validity and reliability of the House-Tree-Person technique remains to be fully demonstrated, this assessment instrument appears to hold promise for use with hearing-impaired adults to anticipate and intervene with potential personality difficulties" (p. 217).

DESIRABLE FEATURES:

The HTP incorporated chromatic as well as achromatic features as part of the assessment. Guidelines for interpretation were clearly demarcated. Also, Buck (1987) provided case examples that illustrated the quantitative and qualitative scoring methods. The manual was very detailed in its approach to design, administration, scoring, and interpretation.

UNDESIRABLE FEATURES:

The quantitative method of the test was quite involved and may take the therapist some time in determining scores. The use of a stopwatch to time the client can be cumbersome. Since the administrator was required to track a myriad of details during the assessment, important data may be missed. It seemed that the client may be prone to exhaustion after completing the drawings as well as the PDI. Interrupting the drawing tasks with a verbal component may interfere with the chromatic version of the test. The way the instructions were worded may develop drawing anxiety in some clients. Additionally, the directions indicated that the drawing should be produced for the administrator. This may promote transference issues that may influence the manner in which the assessment was completed.

OVERALL EVALUATION:

Reliability and validity evidence has yet to be established for the HTP. Some interrater reliability evidence was provided in the pilot studies; yet, they used their own scoring techniques as opposed to the one outlined by Buck (1987). From the studies presented, validity evidence appears mixed. With the quantitative method of scoring the HTP, validity evidence can be established by correlating the results of the HTP with well known standardized measures of intelligence. Additionally, validity evidence can be produced by researching how the HTP distinguishes between clinical populations and well adjusted individuals.

Buck (1987) recommended that the HTP be used as a screening device to measure maladjustment, appraise personality integration, and identify common personality characteristics of a specific population; yet, he did not provide evidence that the HTP was a valid device for screening in these areas. Additionally, he stated that the HTP can be used for employment and placement purposes. If the HTP was to be used to determine job classification decisions, evidence of differential prediction among job positions should be documented (AERA, APA, NCME, 1985). Validity and reliability evidence is required before the HTP can be used as a method of employment or academic placement.

Several questions arise when viewing the standardization sample. First, the population was examined in the late forties. Can this information be used as a reliable guide for interpreting HTP IQs today? The exact nature of classification was not clear. How were these individuals rated? What assessment was used to measure their intelligence level? Was the same assessment used for all subjects? The same questions hold true for the clinical sample. It is not clear how the subjects were labeled and who was responsible for the diagnostic classification. Caution should be taken when using the HTP as a measure of intellectual functioning.

Buck (1987) was very thorough when outlining the administration and scoring sections of the manual. The case illustrations were helpful in providing insight on the use of the HTP. Another positive function of this assessment was that it incorporated color, a factor neglected by some art therapy tests. Future editions of the manual should include more information on the normative sample or develop new norms. Additionally, validity and reliability evidence would be welcome.

REFERENCES

American Educational Research Association, American Psychological Association, & National Council on Measurement in Education. (1985). *Standards for educational and psychological testing.* Washington, DC: American Psychological Association.

Buck, J.N. (1987). *The House-Tree-Person Technique: Revised Manual.* Los Angeles, CA: Western Psychological Services.

Buck, J.N. (1949). The H–T–P technique. *Journal of Clinical Psychology, 5,* 37–74.

Catell, R.B. (1962). *Handbook supplement for Form C of the Sixteen Personality Factor Questionnaire.* Champaign, IL: Institute for Personality and Ability Testing.

Greenson, R. (1967). *The technique and practice of psychoanalysis.* New York: International Universities Press.

Kline, P., and Svaste-Xuto, B. (1981). The House, Tree, Person Test (HTP) in Thailand with 4 and 5 year old children: A comparison of Thai and British results. *Projective Psychology, 26(1),* 1–11.

Lewis, M.L., and Goldstein, M.A. (1981). The use of objectively scorable House-Tree-Person indicators to establish child abuse. *Journal of Clinical Psychology, 37(3),* 667–673.

Marzolf, S.S., and Kirchner, J.H. (1972). House-Tree-Person drawings and personality traits. *Journal of Personality Assessment, 36(2),* 148–165.

Ouellette, S.E. (1988). The use of projective drawing techniques in the personality assessment of prelingually deafened young adults: A pilot study. *A.A.D., July,* 212–217.

Ramirez, C. (1983). Drawing out resistance: The use of the House-Tree-Person Test to facilitate communication in verbal therapy groups. *Group, 7(3),* 39–49.

Teillard, A. (1951). *II Symbolismo del Sogri.* Milan: Feltrineilli. Cited in Ramirez (1983).

Chapter 7

KINETIC HOUSE–TREE–PERSON TEST

TITLE:	Kinetic House-Tree-Person Test (KHTP)
AGE:	age limit not discussed
YEAR:	1987
PURPOSE:	designed to understand human development: Individual transformation process, reflections of self, and relationship to the environment; scoring was based on the presence or absence of attachments and figures
SCORES:	scores included Attachments Present, Figures Other than Self Present, and Additional Figures Present
MANUAL:	manual (213 pages); illustrations (47 pages); profile (5 pages); reliability data (none reported); validity data (none reported)
TIME LIMIT:	no time limit for administration
COST:	$31.95 for testing manual
AUTHOR:	Burns, Robert C.
PUBLISHER:	Brunner/Mazel, Inc., 19 Union Square, New York, NY, 10003.

INTRODUCTION:

Because of the limitations of the House-Tree-Person Test (HTP) and the Draw a Person Test (DAP), researchers moved toward the development of kinetic assessments. "Projective, nonkinetic techniques are criticized because they restrict the depiction of important family dynamics that provide the greatest insight into a child's feelings and perceptions, and his family's roles, influences, and interactions" (Knoff & Prout, 1985, p. 51). One assessment that incorporated a kinetic component was the Kinetic House-Tree-Person Test (KHTP).

As opposed to the HTP, the KHTP combined all three images, house, tree, and person, on one page. In addition, the drawing introduced physical activity of family members. Despite the clinical value of the HTP, Burns (1987; p. 5) remarked on a few limitations:

1. The HTP was standardized on patients in a psychiatric setting.

Literature on the HTP focused on diagnostic labeling such as "Organics, Schizophrenics, etc."

2. Placement of the images occurred on separate pieces of paper that did not allow for action or interaction.

3. Interpretation of the HTP was Freudian and reduced all images to fit within this matrix.

The KHTP was developed to surpass some of the limitations presented by the HTP which resulted in more clinical information about the client.

PURPOSE AND RECOMMENDED USE:

The purpose of the KHTP was to furnish information on the parameters of a client's perspective that may otherwise remain illusive using some traditional drawing techniques such as the HTP. "The K–H–T–P is useful in understanding the dynamics in many types of clinical situations, thus enhancing the healing process" (Burns, 1987, p. 7). The KHTP assessment was devised to tell a story; to create a visual metaphor about self.

DIMENSIONS THAT THE TEST PURPORTS TO MEASURE:

Burns (1987) linked the KHTP to a developmental model, Maslow's (1954) Hierarchy of Needs, to qualitatively measure the results of this assessment. The first five levels of Maslow's (1954) Hierarchy were used to interpret the developmental stages of the person, tree, and house images. Essentially, the house represented the physical aspects of the client's life, the tree indicated life energy and direction, and the person symbolized the client. For instance, Level 1: Belonging to life revealed desire for life, survival, safety, and rootedness. In the drawing of the house, Level 1 was concerned with survival or the desire to die. Approachers viewed the house as a place of security and safety. Access was limited and the house was often depicted as a prison structure. Avoiders were people who considered death. The house may be crumbling, decaying, vacuous or impermanent. In the tree drawings, approachers drew trees that had talon-shaped roots. The tree may appear unfriendly and unclimbable. Avoiders drew trees that were dead or dying. Typically, the trunk was narrow and foliage was absent or sparse. In person drawings, approachers tended to sketch people with an aggressive appearance or paranoid features. The figures were armed and/or suspicious. Avoiders depicted vacuous faces or sad expressions. People seem dead or self-destructive.

ADMINISTRATION:

Using a sheet of $8^{1}/2 \times 11$ inch white paper placed horizontally, the client was asked to "Draw a house, a tree, and a whole person on this piece of paper with some kind of action. Try to draw a whole person, not a cartoon or stick person" (Burns, 1987, p. 5). Group administration, administration qualifications, and test requirements for special populations were not discussed.

NORM GROUPS:

The manual contained several case examples, but the assessment was not standardized on a population. Regardless of Burns' (1987) complaint that the HTP was standardized on a psychiatric population, the KHTP was not standardized on any population. The manner in which the cases were selected remains unclear. Most of the cases appeared to come from a psychiatric population so that the interpretation of drawings made by more well adjusted individuals may be difficult.

INTERPRETATION OF SCORES:

The KHTP was scored for the presence or absence of attachments. For instance, the therapist may observe if the house attached to the tree (H–T) or if the house attached to the person (H–P). Other combinations included the person attached to the tree (P–T), all items attached (H–T–P), or no attachments (None). The KHTP can be scored for figures other than self. For instance, the counselor may record the presence of an antihero, deceased person, parent, friend, hero, relative, unknown person, or other person. Other than summarizing the presence or absence of these items, no other scoring information was discussed.

SOURCE OF ITEMS:

The items appeared to originate from the HTP (Buck, 1948). Using other researchers as a guide, Burns (1987) interpreted the meaning of images drawn on the KHTP. For instance, emphasis of chimneys was said to suggest concern with psychological warmth at home (Buck, 1948; Jolles, 1964) and sexual concern about masculinity (Buck, 1948; Jolles, 1964; Hammer, 1969). Burns (1987) also expressed that emphasis of the chimney suggested concern about power and/or concern about activating creativity; yet, the source of these items remains unclear. Overall, Burns (1987) appeared to draw on the work of previous researchers when discussing interpretation of the objects drawn.

VALIDITY AND RELIABILITY AS DETERMINED BY THE AUTHOR:

Burns (1987) did not incorporate reliability or validity information in his book. He mentioned that kinetic drawings have been reliably scored (Burns & Kaufman, 1972; Knoff & Prout, 1985); yet, he did not provide further information. To date, reliability and validity for the KHTP has not been examined. Although the KHTP was based on the HTP, it cannot be expected to rely on the research used to support the HTP. Additional research was necessary in order to confirm that the KHTP was a reliable and valid art therapy assessment.

DESIRABLE FEATURES:

The test was easy to administer. Further, the manual was easy to read and included several case examples to assist the therapist with interpretation. Adding a kinetic component was a valuable idea. Moving figures will yield more information about personality as compared to static figures. Additionally, combining the house, tree, and person all on one page produces more information than when viewed separately. For instance, when the tree was leaning slightly away from the house, this may indicate growing independence and moving away from family attachments (Burns, 1987). Another possibility was having a person attached to the house. This may suggest a need for nurturing (Burns, 1987). By viewing the interaction of these objects, the therapist was able to glean more information than viewing the house, tree, and person separately.

Not only were attachments and proximity important, but the order in which the items were drawn may reveal information about the client's personality. When the client draws the tree first, it may reveal that "life energy and growth are most important to the drawer. This was typical of people trying to grow or stay alive" (Burns, 1987, p. 102). If the client draws the house first, it may show a need to belong to the earth (a place to survive), need to belong to the body (body needs or obsessions), a need to belong to society, a home for nurturing, or a home for giving and receiving nurturing (Burns, 1987). If the client draws the person first, it may suggest concern with control of feelings, showing off or hiding the body, showing success, a nurturing person, or a joyful person.

Another desirable feature of the KHTP was the incorporation of Maslow's (1954) theory to create a developmental model for the assessment. Burns (1987) modified Maslow's approach to interpret the items on the KHTP. He came up with the following five levels (p. 54):

Level 1: Belong to Life: Desire for life, survival, safety, rootedness.

Level 2: Belong to body: Acceptance of body, seeking control of body addictions and potential.

Level 3: Belong to society: Search for status, success, respect, and power.

Level 4: Belong to self and not-self: Self now defined to include not-self as a pregnant woman accepts her child; compassion, nurturing, giving love; meta motivation.

Level 5: Belong to all living things: Giving and accepting love; self-actualization; sense of good fortune and luck; creativity; celebration of life.

Burns interpreted each item on the KHTP within this framework. Further, he divided each level into Approachers and Avoiders. Burns (1987) provided a similar breakdown for the developmental levels of the tree and person. Also, he included several examples of drawings to indicate the various stages of development.

Burns (1987) also presented an appendix that summarized the general characteristics of the images drawn. These were hypotheses used when judging projective drawing techniques: They involved pressure factors, line or stroke characteristics, drawing size, and placement of the drawing.

For instance, if a drawing was placed low on the page, it was said to suggest feelings of insecurity (Buck, 1948; Jolles, 1964; Burns & Kaufman, 1972), feelings of inadequacy (Buck, 1948; Jolles, 1964; Hammer, 1971; Burns & Kaufman, 1972), or depressive tendencies (Buck, 1948; Machover, 1949; Jolles, 1964; Hammer, 1971). Burns (1987) also furnished a summary of individual characteristics of the house, tree, and person.

UNDESIRABLE FEATURES:

The KHTP may be difficult to interpret when a symbol occurs that was not included in the case examples or the summary tables. For instance, I had one client who drew her person in the shape of a mandala, with two legs, and several eyes. It was not clear how to interpret this figure or where to place it within the developmental model presented by Burns (1987).

Although Burns (1987) provided a table for the scoring of attachments, he did not include scoring information when presenting the case examples. These tables were simplified in that they only note the presence of attachments and figures. Their significance was not discussed. For instance, I would have liked more information on clients who included deceased persons or political figures in their drawings. Obviously, these figures were important; yet, Burns (1987) did not present a framework for interpretation.

OVERALL EVALUATION:

Many have argued about the universal interpretation of symbols. Whether archetypes or cultural symbols, interpretation without the client's input was not valid. Burns warned against the over interpretation of drawing symbols.

> Interpretation of all symbols depends on the level of consciousness of the producer of the symbol at the time the symbol was produced and the level of consciousness of the interpreter at the time of interpretation. There is obviously room for a great deal of error. (Burns, 1987, p. 143)

With this thought in mind, Burns suggested a procedure for interpreting symbols based on level of consciousness. For example, water can have various meanings depending on the consciousness level (p. 147):

Level 1: Survival, embryonic stage

Level 2: "Juices flowing," hedonistic

Level 3: "Power of sea", water beats rock

Level 4: Nurturing, refreshing, useful

Level 5: Flexible, humble, serene, calm

This breakdown was provided for only a few of the symbols. It was not clear how the counselor would use this breakdown when other symbols were present. This point addressed the main weakness of the manual: The interpretation of symbols or drawing features that were not presented by Burns (1987). Granted, the client was the source for interpreting all symbols but what if the client was nonverbal or was unable to communicate the meaning of the item? Regardless of this weakness, the KHTP yielded some valuable information about the client's perception of herself, the environment, and her family. The kinetic component was a valuable addition to the HTP. The interaction of the items as well as the developmental model were a strong improvement over the HTP.

Overall, the manual was clear and the test was easy to administer. Additional research information was needed on this assessment, especially the reliability and validity of symbol interpretation. Also, it would be interesting to have information on the chromatic version of the test. Color choice may reveal additional information about the client. The investigation of possible cultural differences that may be found in the KHTP would be worthwhile.

REFERENCES

Buck, J.N. (1948). *The House-Tree-Person Technique.* Los Angeles, CA: Western Psychological Services.

Burns, R.C. (1987). *Kinetic-House-Tree-Person-Drawings: An interpretive manual.* New York, NY: Brunner/Mazel.

Burns, R.C., and Kaufman, S.H. (1972). *Actions, styles and symbols in kinetic family drawings (K–F–D): An interpretive manual.* New York: Brunner/Mazel.

Hammer, E.F. (1969). Hierarchical organization of personality and the H–T–P, achromatic and chromatic. In Buck, J.N., and Hammer, E.F. (Eds.) *Advances in the House-Tree-Person Techniques: Variations and Applications.* Los Angeles, CA: Western Psychological Services.

Hammer, E.F. (1971). *The clinical application of projective drawings.* Springfield, IL: Charles C Thomas.

Jolles, I. (1964). *A catalog for the qualitative interpretation of the House-Tree-Person (H–T–P).* Los Angeles, CA: Western Psychological Services.

Knoff, H.M., and Prout, H.T. (1985). The kinetic drawing system: A review and integration of the Kinetic Family and School Drawing techniques. *Psychology in the Schools, 22 (January),* 50–59.

Machover, K. (1949). *Personality projection in the drawing of the human figure.* Springfield, IL: Charles C Thomas.

Maslow, A.H. (1954). *Motivation and personality.* New York: Harper and Row.

Chapter 8

FAMILY–CENTERED CIRCLE DRAWINGS

TITLE: Family-Centered Circle Drawings (FCCD)
AGE: age limit not discussed
YEAR: 1990
PURPOSE: designed to understand parent-self relationships
SCORES: drawings were not scored; guidelines for interpretation were presented; four types of FCCDs: (1) Mother-centered; (2) Father-centered; (3) Self-centered; and (4) Parent-self-centered
MANUAL: manual (198 pages); illustrations (49 pages); profile (12 pages); reliability data (none reported); validity data (none reported)
TIME LIMIT: no time limit for administration
COST: $29.95 for testing manual
AUTHOR: Burns, Robert C.
PUBLISHER: Brunner/Mazel, Inc., 19 Union Square, New York, NY, 10003.

INTRODUCTION:

Family-Centered Circle Drawings (FCCD; Burns, 1990) were based on the concept of inner parents and the relationship to the self. Through the creation of symbol systems in drawings, therapists may determine how clients relate to their parents. Specifically, clients' emotions towards their parents and barriers between them were discussed in comparison to the clients' inner parents. Since symbol systems were created by the client, they were unique and served to bring the person closer to center (Burns, 1990).

FCCDs were based partly on Rorschach's findings relating to increased projective material with symmetry. Although standardized inkblot tests were previously used, Rorschach (1942) was the first to apply inkblots to assessment of personality as a whole (Anastasi, 1988). Rorschach (1942) discovered that symmetrical inkblots produced more responses and more unconscious material than asymmetrical inkblots. Burns (1990) incorporated this research by placing individual family members in a centered, symmetrical matrix. By drawing parents and self, the client may begin to see parent-self relationships more clearly and the impact on her own inner parents.

Jung's work with mandalas also contributed to the FCCD. According to Burns (1990), a mandala was a centered symbol in a symmetrical design.

> Psychologically speaking, a mandala image is one that emphasizes the totality of something, usually showing quite clearly a periphery and a center. In its historical sense, the term mandala refers to certain very structured meditation symbols used in Buddhism, often consisting of a four-gated square or circular city with a central image (to be meditated on) and lesser images surrounding it. (Hall, 1983, p. 76)

Jung extensively studied mandalas in his search for balance and health (Coward, 1985). Additionally, Jung was a novice artist who worked through his own conflicts by painting and sculpting: "In fact, Jung's theories can best be understood in the context of the value he attached to the subjective reality of spontaneously generated images" (Rubin, 1987, p. 93). The FCCD combined the use of the mandala with the concept of centering and artistic expression. Burns (1990) perceived that the key to these drawings was centering:

> By centering a symbol and focusing upon it in a symmetrical matrix, one may elicit deep emotional reactions. In the religious world focusing upon centered symbols such as a cross, star, lamb, divine figure, and so on may bring insights and healing. In the projective drawing world, centering upon the self-created images of the parents or of the parents and the self may also bring insights and healing. (Burns, 1990, p. 2)

By placing family figures in the center of the circle, Burns (1990) believed that it would increase projective material. Using this approach, the therapist fostered a dialogue with the client's inner parents in order to determine barriers and emotional conflicts.

PURPOSE AND RECOMMENDED USE:

The purpose of the FCCD was to gain information about the client's family and relate it to the client's view of self and her inner parents. According to Burns (1990), this technique allowed the client to see herself more clearly in relationship to each parent. Positive and negative associations were made around the symbols systems that the client created. The FCCD was recommended for those clients who need to get in touch with their inner parents. The objective of Burns' (1990) approach was to furnish counselors with an awareness of the client's visual communication potential. Also, therapists may be able to provide a broader interpretive context that was not heavily dependent on verbal skills.

DIMENSIONS THAT THE TEST PURPORTS TO MEASURE:

The FCCD incorporated four types of drawings: (1) Mother-centered, (2) Father-centered, (3) Self-centered, and (4) Parent-self-centered. Each drawing generated information about the client's perception of family and self. The FCCD began by placing one parent in the center of a circle while the client free associated, doodled, or drew symbols around the perimeter of the circle. The FCCD was repeated with the parent of the opposite sex, and then with the self at the center of the circle. Parents-self-centered drawings (PSCD) involved placing both parents and self in the center circle. The client then free associated images around the circle. Symbol-Centered Probes (SYMCP) focused on one particular symbol from the FCCD or PSCD. The client placed this symbol in the circle and then free associated images around this object. In turn, this generated additional information regarding client issues.

ADMINISTRATION:

All drawings were to be completed on a standard sheet of typing paper 8½ by 11 inches with the circle already drawn on the paper. The diameter of the circle ranged from 7½ to 9 inches. Three separate drawings were obtained for the FCCD. The instructions were as follows:

> Draw your mother in the center of a circle. Visually free associate with drawn symbols around the periphery of the circle. Try to draw a whole person, not a stick or cartoon figure. (Burns, 1990, p. 3)

This procedure was repeated substituting the father and then the self for the mother. The instructions were similar for the PSCD. For younger or educationally limited clients, Burns (1990) substituted the following instructions:

> Draw your parents and yourself in the middle of a circle. Try to draw whole

people, not stick people or cartoons. Doodle whatever you want around the edge of the circle. (Burns, 1990, p. 109)

Other requirements for administration were not discussed, such as the administrator's qualifications, drawing media choices, group administration, or use with special populations.

NORM GROUPS:

The FCCD was not standardized on a population. Burns (1990) used the case approach and presented example drawings with limited information on the client's background. The manner in which these clients were selected was unclear. Generally, the cases represented a clinical population. People dealing with eating disorders, addictive disorders, or family violence were just a few of the client issues. Although Burns (1990) posed a list of qualities seen in well adjusted individuals, only one drawing was included. No background information was presented on the person who drew the "healthy" PSCD.

INTERPRETATION OF SCORES:

Burns (1990) included a list of items to observe in an FCCD. For instance, the therapist should observe the size of the figure since it was often a reflection of the psychological size and the amount of energy invested in the figure. The omission or overemphasis of body parts and facial expressions should be considered. Also, the therapist should determine whether symbols surrounding the self were repeated in the parental drawings. Symbols directly above a figure should be noted since they were associated with primary feelings. For instance, a knife drawn above a figure may suggest anger (Burns, 1990). The positive and/or negative tone of the symbols should be observed. Although Burns (1990) admitted that these were just a few items to observe, further guidelines for interpretation were not provided. Similar instructions were included for the PSCD. In the last chapter, Burns (1990) discussed a list of qualities observed in maladjusted individuals compared to a list of characteristics viewed in healthy people. The appendix contained recurring symbols in Kinetic Family Drawings (KFD) and FCCD that Burns (1990) considered important. The following represented a few examples from the appendix:

Butterflies: This symbol is associated with the search for illusive love and beauty.

Drums: A symbol found in the drawings for those who have difficulty in expressing anger openly and thus displace their anger onto the drum.

The instructions did not note the manner in which the drawing was completed, the client's affect during the drawing, or type of media used.

SOURCE OF ITEMS:

The source of the circle drawings was previously discussed. Burns (1990) based his approach on Freud's work with free association, Jung's work with mandalas, and Rorschach's work with the standardized ink-blot test. The source of the interpretation of common symbols was ambiguous. For instance, the list of items in the appendix incorporated interpretations for various symbols. It was not clear if this list represented Burns (1990s) interpretations or the interpretations based on the work of previous researchers.

VALIDITY AND RELIABILITY
AS DETERMINED BY THE AUTHOR:

Burns (1990) did not investigate the reliability or validity of the FCCD. Also, he did not use a population to standardize this assessment. The validity of the items in the appendix was questionable. The test manual did not include many examples of children's or adolescents' work. Most of the clients were in their thirties and forties. Other demographic characteristics of the clients were not presented. Whether the FCCD was a valid and reliable instrument for children or adults was unclear. It would be interesting to collect data on the interpretations of a variety of practitioners such as art therapists, counselors, and psychologists to see if there was reliable agreement among professionals. To date, no research was available that examined the reliability and validity of this assessment.

DESIRABLE FEATURES:

The FCCD was an interesting assessment in that it provided information about the client with respect to his/her parents. It was different from the Kinetic Family Drawing (KFD; Burns & Kaufman, 1972) in that the therapist was able to see the client's relationship with one parent at a time and focus in on one particular symbol. When I implemented the FCCD in private practice, the client gained insight from the types of symbols that were drawn in relation to self and to his/her parents. This assessment seemed to be more helpful in uncovering the barriers in the client's past relationship with his/her parents as opposed to discovering or getting in touch with their inner parents.

UNDESIRABLE FEATURES:

Burns (1990) did not outline what types of drawing media the administrator should make available to the client. It was difficult to tell from the drawings included in the book what type of medium was used and if it was consistently used. The addition of color may significantly affect the outcome of the assessment; yet, this was not addressed by Burns (1990).

Interpretation of the FCCD appeared limited. It focused only on the drawing and neglected other aspects of the domain. For instance, observing a client's affect while drawing yielded important information. In addition, the manner in which something was drawn or erased may be significant to the interpretation of the drawing. Some may consider the FCCD a "cookbook" approach (Koppitz, 1968). Burns' (1990) FCCD did not contain a list of symbols that the counselor looks up for interpretation. Much of the interpretation was left up to the client which has a positive function. Yet, it did follow the cookbook approach to art therapy in that it neglected to observe the manner in which the drawings were completed. Valuable information regarding client affect may be missed if the therapist did not observe the drawing process.

OVERALL EVALUATION:

Burns (1990) combined free association, family of origin work, object relations, and Jungian mandala symbolism to create an assessment that helped the client view herself in relationship to her parents and her inner parents. Through a series of centered circle drawings, the client created a visual dialog about her relationships with her family. The book contained many examples of each of these drawings.

Although Burns (1990) provided large collection of drawings and explained how to create them, they were in black and white. The colors and media used were not discussed. Thus, the reader lacks a complete visual sense of the drawings. Paint, pastels, inks, and watercolors were some of the materials that clients can manipulate when creating art. Texture of the material was often a reflection of the artist's inner experience or feelings:

> As one avenue to self-definition, we have usually had some choice of art materials, and have on occasion asked that people define themselves by choosing to be an art medium or process, and sharing their reasons. We have found that their choice is intimately related to how they see themselves, i.e., soft or hard, flexible or firm, fragile or strong, colorful or bland, etc. The choice of medium then evolves into a productive activity with that medium, in both cases self-defining and enhancing self-awareness. (Moreno, 1975, p. 113)

Art therapists use the characteristics of art materials for diagnostic purposes. For instance, watercolors involve complex layering. This medium was unpredictable and transparent in nature that allowed the artist spontaneous expression. Since watercolors were hard to control, Robbins (1987) stressed that people who employ this medium were spontaneous individuals who accepted change and relinquished omnipotence. Working with oils was a time consuming process because it entailed layering. People who used this medium were patient, allowed change, and preferred a predetermined challenge (Robbins, 1987). The use of pencil indicated a need for control, structure, and firm boundaries (Robbins, 1987). Finger paint was a direct form of expression. Betensky (1973) described finger paint as an agent of regression that provided an important outlet for stress. These were just a few examples of media as they related to personality characteristics. Although painting may not be an appropriate medium for this assessment, the choice of color would be revealing. For instance, a client may use colored pencils, oil pastels, or crayons to create his FCCD.

Additional information was needed regarding the reliability and validity of the FCCD. It was an interesting approach that revealed information about the client's relationship with self and family; yet, the assessment lacked important data regarding administration requirements, interpretation, and a norm population. Research on the relationship between the KFD and the FCCD would be beneficial. One advantage of the KFD was that it observed sibling systems. Sibling interactions greatly effect the dynamics of the family system. "There is a high level of interaction among siblings in the home and that the quality of this interaction is rich and varied" (Abramovitch et al., p. 1003). In my private practice, Burns' (1990) approach was modified to include siblings. This disclosed important information about the client's relationship issues. The validity and reliability of varying Burns' (1990) approach should be examined.

Also, it would be helpful to have more information on the use of the FCCD with children and special populations such as learning disabled, hearing impaired, and culturally diverse individuals. Overall, the FCCD had great potential as an art therapy assessment. With additional research information, the FCCD may be a valuable tool when viewing the client's relationship to herself and her family.

REFERENCES

Abramovitch, R., Corter, C., and Lando, B. (1979). Sibling interaction in the home. *Child Development, 50,* 997–1003.

Anastasi, A. (1988). *Psychological testing.* 6th ed. New York: Macmillian.

Betensky, M. (1973). *Self-discovery through self-expression: Use of art in psychotherapy.* Springfield, IL: Charles C Thomas.

Burns, R.C. (1990). *A guide to family-centered circle drawings.* New York: Brunner/Mazel.

Burns, R.C., and Kaufman, S.H. (1972). *Actions, styles, and symbols in Kinetic Family Drawings (K–F–D): An interpretive manual.* New York: Brunner/Mazel.

Coward, H. (1985). *Jung and eastern thought.* New York: State University of New York Press.

Hall, J.A. (1983). *Jungian dream interpretation: A Handbook of theory and practice.* Toronto, Canada: Inner City Books.

Koppitz, E.M. (1968). *Psychological evaluation of children's human figure drawings.* New York: Grune & Stratton.

Moreno, Z.T. (1975). *Group psychotherapy and psychodrama.* New York: Beacon House.

Robbins, A. (1987). *The artist as therapist.* New York: Human Sciences Press.

Rorschach, H. (1942). *Psychodiagnostics.* Berne: Verlag Has Huber.

Rubin, J.A. (1987). *Approaches to art therapy.* New York: Brunner/Mazel.

Chapter 9

SILVER DRAWING TEST

TITLE: Silver Drawing Test (SDT)
AGE: ages five and over
YEAR: 1990
PURPOSE: designed to assess cognitive abilities in three areas: sequential concepts, spatial concepts, and association and formation of concepts; also designed to screen for depression
SCORES: five scores included Predictive Drawing, Drawing from Observation, Drawing from Imagination, Total, and Projection (Emotional Content)
MANUAL: manual (92 pages); profile (11 pages); reliability data (8 pages); validity data (13 data pages)
TIME LIMIT: 10–20 minutes for administration
COST: $39.95 for testing manual, 10 test booklets, 10 scoring forms, and layout sheet
AUTHOR: Silver, Rawley
PUBLISHER: Albin Press Distributors; 3332 Hadfield Greene, Sarasota, FL 34235.

INTRODUCTION:

The Silver Drawing Test (SDT; 1990) was one of the few art therapy assessments that was written according to the Standards for Educational and Psychological Testing (AERA, APA, NCME, 1985). Silver (1990) provided information on the theoretical background of the assessment, normative information, reliability, and validity studies. Although Silver (1990) discussed research evidence, the SDT had several weaknesses.

PURPOSE AND RECOMMENDED USE:

The SDT measured a person's cognitive skills and adjustment. Additionally, it was purported to be a screening device for depression.

According to Silver (1990), the SDT had four goals: (1) to bypass language in assessing the ability to solve conceptual problems; (2) to provide precision in evaluating cognitive strengths or weaknesses that may not be detected by verbal measures; (3) to facilitate identification of children or adolescents who may be depressed; and (4) to provide a pre-post instrument for assessing the effectiveness of therapeutic or educational programs. By detecting low levels of cognitive development and depression, the SDT aided in determining individuals in need of new educational programs and/or counseling. Silver (1990) designed the SDT based on the premise that drawings can be used to identify and evaluate problem solving capabilities.

> Children's drawings are pictorial devices that can represent reality vicariously and economically, and thus reflect their thinking. Children with inadequate language ability are deprived of many opportunities to represent their experiences because they lack a major device for constructing models of reality. (Silver, 1990, p. 9)

The SDT was designed to assess cognitive abilities and depression for children and adults. The test manual reported that individual or group administration was appropriate. For children under seven or people who had difficulty understanding directions, individual administration was recommended (Silver, 1990). Individual administration was also recommended in clinical settings to allow for discussion and behavioral observation.

DIMENSIONS THAT THE TEST PURPORTS TO MEASURE:

The SDT measured the individual's cognition in the following areas: (1) Predictive Drawing; (2) Drawing from Observation; and (3) Drawing from Imagination. The Predictive Drawing subtest evaluated sequencing abilities. In addition, this subtest assessed the ability to deal with hypothetical situations involving conservation. The Drawing from Observation subtest evaluated concepts of space particularly, horizontal, vertical, and depth reasoning. The ability to form concepts was assessed in the Drawing from Imagination subtest. Specifically, the skills of selecting, combining, and representing objects was tested. Also, the emotional content of the drawing was noted.

ADMINISTRATION:

Generally, the SDT took about 10 to 20 minutes to complete. The test can be administered individually or in groups with no limit on time. Silver (1990) recommended that group administration of the test was not appropriate for children below age seven and for those people who had difficulty understanding directions. For individuals who had difficulty reading, oral administration was recommended. The SDT was standardized in the English language. Although Silver (1990) purported that the test can be used with hearing impaired children, guidelines were not discussed for working with this population or other culturally diverse groups.

According to Silver (1990), the SDT can be administered and scored by teachers, therapists, or psychologists; yet, she did not know if training was necessary. No other administration requirements were discussed. Reliability values for the different methods of administration were not discussed.

NORM GROUPS:

The SDT norms were developed from 547 students in grades 1 to 12 in rural, urban, and suburban schools. Grades 6, 7, 9, and 11 were not clearly represented. Although grade 6 does appear in the normative information, the students from this grade were grouped together with fourth and fifth graders with a N of 36. The students came from 13 different schools representing the low to middle socioeconomic backgrounds. Other demographic characteristics of the sample were not discussed. A population of hearing impaired students was not represented.

The SDT for adults was standardized on 77 adults. Silver (1990) stated that 250 workshop participants, including undergraduate students, graduate students, social workers, therapists, teachers, and parents of handicapped children took the SDT from which 20 subjects were randomly selected. Apparently the remainder of the normative information came from undergraduate and graduate students in three different states. The method of selection for this part of the sample did not appear to be random. The cultural background of the subjects was not discussed. No other information on the demographics of the standardization sample was presented. It was not clear how the samples were selected or randomized. The adult standardization sample was clearly a restricted sample and not representative of the general population. Sex differences were not examined for either group. Essentially, there was no evidence of a well-defined norm group for adults or children.

INTERPRETATION OF SCORES:

Scores were expressed as percentile ranks and T-scores. Tables 24 and 25 provided total and subscale scores. Grades 9 and 11 were missing from these tables and Silver (1990) did not provide instructions to the administrator concerning score interpretation. Apparently, individuals in grades 9 and 11 can have two scores, one above their grade level and one below. Tables were provided for the classifications of subscale scores for each form of the test using the same grade levels. As with the previous tables, the manual did not state how the cutoff points were determined. With the exception of scoring a 9th or 11th grader's SDT, the tables were easy to use.

Initially, Silver (1990) stated that hearing impaired children differed in the cognitive abilities as compared to hearing children. Yet, Silver (1990) did not provide a normative sample of hearing impaired children. Additionally, the scoring procedures for this populations were not discussed. This remained true for learning disabled and culturally diverse populations. Without demographic information on the normative sample, users of the SDT should be cautioned when working with culturally diverse populations.

SOURCE OF ITEMS:

How the drawing exercises were selected was unclear. The method of selection and criteria were not presented. Also the people who selected the items and their qualifications were not discussed. Not only was the source of the items unclear, the nature of the items used to screen for depression was unclear. There was no mention in the manual how the items were designated as depression screeners. The criteria for item selection, both for the subscale categories and depression, were not presented in the test manual. This lack of evidence did not provide support for the content validity of the test.

VALIDITY AS DETERMINED BY THE AUTHOR:

Content validity evidence, which was discussed previously, was lacking. As to criterion related validity, the manual reported correlations of .33, .16, .37, and .29 between the three SDT subtest scores and the total score with the WISC Performance Scale. WISC verbal correlations were near zero. Also, SDT subtest scores ranged from .59, .37, .50, and .60 with WAIS. Correlations with Draw a Man Test were .75, .31, .62, and .72. Correlations with the Bender were negative. Overall, concurrent validity was mixed. As for the achievement measures correlations, they were very low, which may suggest discriminate validity. Yet, with aptitude measures, correlations were too low to indicate convergence.

When evaluating the correlations of the subtests, one category stood out: Drawing from Observation which consistently received very low correlations (ranging from −.15 to .47), most of which were not significant. The validity of this subtest was highly questionable. In addition, Predictive Drawing received the second lowest correlations, ranging from .16 to .36, most of which were not significant. Very little information was provided by Silver (1990) on how the data were collected. Inconsistencies in data collection were mentioned. For example, she used the Otis Lennon Test for most children, yet used school records for test scores of deaf and learning disabled children. Since the Otis Lennon Test was not administered to this population, their scores should have been separated out. The only group Silver (1990) separated out was a group of deaf children and she used WISC Performance Scores to correlate with the SDT.

Missing from all of the validity evidence were correlations with depression indexes. Silver (1990) purported that the SDT can be used as a screening device for depression; yet, she did not provide evidence that the instrument discriminated for depression. Since validity evidence did not exist, the SDT was obviously not an indicator for depression.

RELIABILITY AS DETERMINED BY THE AUTHOR:

In a test-retest study, the SDT was administered to 10 third grade children one month later. Although all the third grade students were initially evaluated, the teacher selected ten "top students across the board." Without a random sample within this population, the reliability information was suspect. Other than coming from lower income families in an urban neighborhood, demographic characteristics were not discussed. Silver (1990) included herself along with four other individuals to score the SDT's. It seemed obvious that she would know how to score the instrument since she designed it; therefore, excluding herself from scoring the instruments would have made the study more objective. The overall probability level was not significant. When viewing the subtests, Predictive Drawing was not significantly reliable for these third grade students. Although Silver (1990) tried to explain what the children did differently, the evidence remained that this section of the test was not a reliable indicator. In addition, using only ten subjects did not lend itself to strong reliability evidence. It was possible that the test may be reliable for only third grade students, not adults, hearing impaired children, or other grade levels.

Silver (1990) cited reliability evidence from Moser (1980). Unfortunately, Silver (1990) did not provide a reference list so that the reader could refer to the original article. I was unable to find information on Moser's (1980) research. According to Silver (1990), Moser (1980) administered the SDT to 12 learning disabled adolescents using a one month interval. Again, demographic information was missing. Moser (1980) found that all subtests were significant yet the reader was not given information on how these correlations were computed. Information on who scored the tests was not presented.

Excluding herself from the study, Silver (1990) used four judges from the previous study to examine the reliability of the Emotional Projection part of the SDT. The result was not significant. She attributed this to lack of practice and misunderstanding the scoring guidelines. Silver (1990) conversed with each judge to clear up any ambiguity and the resulting correlation was significant. Therefore, it appeared that reading the test manual alone was not sufficient for scoring this portion of the test. Without her intervention, the Emotional Projection part of the test was not reliable.

Using one educator, an art therapist, and a psychotherapist, all with no special training, Silver (1990) provided evidence of reliability using herself as a reference. Correlations of the subtests ranged from .45 to .99. The Emotional Projection part of the test was not examined.

RESEARCH USING THE SDT:

At this time, research information on the SDT is not available. I did find Draw-a-Story Test (DAS), by Silver (1988), which was used as a screening device for depression and emotional needs. Although Silver did not refer to the DAS in her manual on the SDT, it provided information about the Drawing from Imagination task. The goals of the DAS were as follows: (1) to identify depressed individuals; (2) to provide access for therapeutic dialogue; and (3) to increase understanding of depressive illness. Silver selected 14 stimulus drawings from 65 drawings used in two previous instruments. How the drawings were selected and who was involved in the selection process remained unclear.

As with the Drawing from Imagination subtest of the SDT, the participant was asked to select two images and make a drawing that tells a story for the DAS. Silver (1988) reported that group and individual administration was possible with this test. It should be noted that only a few of these 14 images appeared in the Drawing from Imagination subtest on the SDT. Interpretation and scoring of the DAS was the same as for the Drawing from Imagination subtest.

Interscorer reliability was reported to be .80 which was significant at the .001 level. Silver (1988) reported that the DAS was a reliable measure yet did not present statistical information. Out of a class of 24 third grade students, she chose 12 to be retested since they responded with negative fantasies. A few questions arose when reading the section on reliability. Why not retest the entire group? How long was the retest interval? What are the demographic characteristics of this population?

Silver (1988) conducted a final study to determine if the DAS can be used as a screening device for depression. A score of one point on the DAS indicated strongly negative themes such as hopelessness and sadness. Silver's (1988) hypothesis was that depressed individuals would score one point on the DAS. Although the subjects were not randomly selected, Silver did include some demographic information. When she tested her hypothesis, she found that only depressed children and adolescents typically scored one point. The results were not significant for depressed adults.

This suggested that the DAS instrument might be useful as a first step in identifying some, but not all, depressed children and adolescents. Although strongly negative responses did not necessarily indicate depression, and conversely, positive responses did not exclude depression, the findings suggested that a child or adolescent who responded with a strongly negative fantasy may be at risk for depression, and that thorough evaluation would be worthwhile. (Silver, 1988, p. 76)

Although the validity of the DAS was not examined and reliability was questionable, it did provide theoretical information about the Drawing from Imagination subtest used in the SDT. It was surprising that even though Silver did not find complete support in using this task as a screening device for depression that she would continue to purport that SDT indicates depression.

DESIRABLE FEATURES:

The SDT can be used with both children, adults, and nonreaders. The test can be administered in group settings or individually. "Its brevity is useful for subjects with histories of limited attention span" (Horovitz, 1985, p. 44). Also, it provided a breakdown of cognitive skills into three different areas: sequential concepts, spatial concepts, and association and formation of concepts. The latter half of the manual was devoted to scoring examples that were helpful to the administrator.

UNDESIRABLE FEATURES:

Although Silver (1990) provided guidelines for scoring the SDT, this may not be enough, as shown by the reliability evidence. A particularly complicated section of the test, Drawing from Observation, would be better understood in the form of a lecture and practice sessions for interpretation prior to administration. Since Drawing from Observation was difficult to interpret, it may partly explain why this portion of the test was not valid nor reliable.

When using the percentile ranks and T-score conversion charts, scores for ninth and eleventh graders were missing. This was confusing since Silver (1990) did not provide information on how to score individuals in these grade levels. This lack of consistency may be an issue when trying to provide evidence for reliability and validity.

OVERALL EVALUATION:

The largest problem with the SDT was the lack of evidence to support the claim that the instrument was a discriminator of depression. Since

Silver (1990) did not even attempt to provide this evidence, the SDT should not be used as an indicator of depression. More importantly, there was no evidence of randomized samples. Since the demographics of the sample, particularly one's cultural background, were not discussed, it was difficult to determine how the results generalize to other populations.

Validity evidence was found lacking for this instrument, particularly the subtest of Drawing from Observation and Predictive Drawing. Silver (1990) neglected to establish validity evidence for the Emotional Projection section of the test. Silver's (1990) rationale for selecting the tests used to correlate with the SDT was not clear.

> Also, many of the table legends are erroneous or misleading. Some of the test titles are listed incorrectly and, in several tables, the N value provided is the sum of all cases, although the data are actually based on several groups. (Crehan, 1989)

Crehan (1989) also noted that, according to Silver's (1990) theoretical foundation, learning disabled children were high in visual-spatial skills, moderate in conceptual skills, and low in sequencing skills; yet, no evidence existed to support this point. The same evidence was lacking for hearing impaired populations.

In sum, content validity was found lacking in that the test specifications were not discussed. It was not clear how the test items were selected. However, discriminate evidence was provided between the SDT and nominal achievement measures. Criterion related validity (predictive) data did not provide evidence of convergence (Crehan, 1989). Criterion related validity (concurrent) was mixed and in some cases so low that one questioned what the SDT may be measuring. Concurrent validity evidence for depression was not discussed.

The SDT was unreliable (Horovitz, 1985). Small sample sizes and ambiguity in scoring procedures limited the reliability information. Interscorer reliability evidence was questionable since Silver (1990) included herself, and in one case, intervened and talked with the judges before conducting a second evaluation of reliability. Content sampling reliability evidence was not discussed.

I agree with previous reviewers (Crehan, 1989; Chase, 1989; and Mealor, 1989) that the SDT was a creative attempt to measure cognitive skills in a nonverbal approach. Yet, there was no evidence to indicate what the test measures or how well it does so. Additional studies, that include demographic information, need to be conducted to establish reliability and validity of this instrument. Normative samples need to be reevaluated. Although most tests were standardized on hearing populations, "norms established on deaf children are useful in a number of situations pertaining to the educational development of these children" (Anastasi, 1988). In order to be used as a screen for depression, Silver (1990) must provide validity evidence, otherwise, the SDT cannot be used as an indicator of depression.

REFERENCES

American Educational Research Association, American Psychological Association, & National Council on Measurement in Education. (1985). *Standards for educational and psychological testing.* Washington, DC: American Psychological Association.

Anastasi, A. (1988). *Psychological testing.* 6th ed. New York: Macmillan.

Chase, C.I. (1989). Review of the Silver Drawing Test of Cognitive and Creative Skills. *Mental Measurements 1989 book.* (10: 745). Lincoln, NE: Burrs Institute of Mental Measurements.

Crehan, K.D. (1989). Review of the Silver Drawing Test of Cognitive Skills and Adjustment. *Mental Measurements 1989 book.* (10: 333). Lincoln, NE: Burrs Institute of Mental Measurements.

Horovitz, E.G. (1985). Silver Drawing Test of Cognitive and Creative Skills. *Art Therapy, March,* p. 44.

Mealor, D.J. (1989). Review of the Silver Drawing Test of Cognitive and Creative Skills. *Mental Measurements 1989 book.* (10: 747). Lincoln, NE: Burrs Institute of Mental Measurements.

Silver, R. (1990). *Silver Drawing Test of Cognitive Skills and Adjustment.* Sarasota, FL: Ablin Press.

Silver, R. (1988). *Draw-a-Story: Screening for depression and emotional needs.* Mamaroneck, NY: Abalone Press.

Chapter 10

DRAW A PERSON TEST

TITLE:	Draw a Person Test: Screening Procedure for Emotional Disturbance (DAP: SPED)
AGE:	for children and adolescents (6 to 17 years)
YEAR:	1991
PURPOSE:	designed to identify individuals who have emotional problems and are in need of further evaluation
SCORES:	yields a standard score which is used to determine if further assessment is (1) not indicated, (2) indicated, or (3) strongly indicated
MANUAL:	manual (71 pages); illustrations (14 pages); profile (4 pages); reliability data (2 pages); validity data (5 pages)
TIME LIMIT:	maximum time limit of 15 minutes for administration
COST:	$29.00 for testing manual; $29.00 for (25) record forms; $64.00 for complete kit
AUTHOR:	Naglieri, Jack A., McNeish, Timothy J., and Bardos, Achilles N.
PUBLISHER:	PRO–ED, 8700 Shoal Creek Boulevard, Austin, TX 78758-6897.

INTRODUCTION:

The Draw a Person Screening Procedure for Emotional Disturbance (DAP: SPED; Naglieri et al., 1991) was developed to serve as an aid in the identification of children or adolescents who may be behaviorally or emotionally disordered. The authors of the DAP: SPED designed a quantitative scoring system that would distinguish between behaviorally disordered and normal populations. Also, the instrument ensued from the Draw A Person: A Quantitative Scoring System (DAP: QSS; Naglieri, 1988) which assessed cognition. Using the DAP: SPED, emotional status and cognitive development can be assessed.

PURPOSE AND RECOMMENDED USE:

The DAP: SPED was planned as a screening procedure used to identify individuals in need of evaluation for emotional problems. The authors reported that the test may be useful in identifying children who suffer from behavioral problems. Additionally, school counselors may use the instrument to identify students in need of individual or group counseling. The authors suggested that the DAP: SPED can be incorporated into the regular psychoeducational assessment battery. The DAP: SPED may be used during initial interviews or initial family assessments. The authors recommended that the DAP: SPED be followed by additional testing and/or referrals to professional agencies.

DIMENSIONS THAT THE TEST PURPORTS TO MEASURE:

The scores of the DAP: SPED were grouped into three categories based on need of additional assessment that (1) is not indicated, (2) is indicated, or (3) is strongly indicated. For example, if a child received a score of less than 55 points, further evaluation for emotional problems was not indicated. If a child received a score of 55 to 64, additional evaluation was indicated. Should a child receive a score of 65 or above, further evaluation was strongly indicated. It was not clear how these cutoff scores were determined. The authors recommended that the cutoff scores should not be rigidly applied.

> Additionally, because we recognize the limitations of any screening approach, we suggest that the users may cautiously apply other criteria depending upon their setting and goals. When doing so, the nature of the DAP: SPED as a screening instrument and the issues involved with setting a cutoff score should be carefully considered. (Naglieri et al., 1991, p. 63)

Forms for rating the cognitive development of the client were included in a separate assessment (DAP: QSS, Naglieri, 1988). The same drawings for the DAP: SPED can be used to rate cognitive development. For additional information on scoring cognition, please refer to the DAP: QSS (Naglieri, 1988).

ADMINISTRATION:

The authors required users of the DAP: SPED to have training and experience in test theory and development, including individual and group assessment procedures. Although qualifications and titles vary from state to state, the authors stated that psychologists, school psychologists, counselors, diagnosticians, behavior specialists, special educational personnel, learning specialists, speech and language specialists, rehabilitation professions, physicians, and social workers have the training to administer, score, and interpret the DAP: SPED.

The DAP: SPED required strict adherence to administration guidelines. The examiner should allow a maximum of five minutes for completion of each drawing. Should the individual finish before five minutes, the examiner should proceed to the next drawing. The following directions were outlined for individual administration:

> I'd like you to draw some pictures for me. First I'd like you to draw a picture of a man. Make the very best picture you can. Take your time and work very carefully, and I'll tell you when to stop. Remember, be sure to draw the whole man. Please begin. (Allow five minutes.)

> This time I want you to draw a picture of a woman. Make the very best picture you can. Take your time and work very carefully, and I'll tell you when to stop. Be sure to draw the whole woman. Please begin. (Allow five minutes.)

> Now I'd like you to draw a picture of yourself. Be sure to draw the very best picture you can. Take your time and work very carefully, and I'll tell you when to stop. Be sure to draw your whole self. Please begin.

The directions for group administration were similar and included the same time constraints. Each examinee should have a pencil with an eraser and a DAP: SPED Record Form. The examiner was responsible for completing the demographic information on the front of the Record Form.

NORM GROUPS:

The DAP: SPED standardization sample was drawn from a population of 4,468 children aged 5 to 17 years. They were the same individuals used to standardize the DAP: QSS (Naglieri, 1988). Using the 1980 census data as a guide, a sample representative of the population in terms of age, gender, geographic region, race, socioeconomic status, and ethnicity was identified. The authors provided tables on the demographic characteristics of the samples including breakdowns by age, gender, geographic region, etc. The authors did an excellent job of providing information on the standardization sample. The resulting sample included 2,260 students from 6 to 17 years of age.

INTERPRETATION OF SCORES:

The scoring system was comprised of two types of items. First, the DAP: SPED included items dealing with figure dimensions. Templates were used for scoring these items. Three sets of three templates, one for each age group 6 to 8, 9 to 12, and 13–17 years), were used for items one through eight. The templates were used to determine the size of the figure, the slant of the figure, and placement on the page. The manual contained clear directions and illustrations that aided in the scoring of these items.

The second group of items dealt with rating the content of the drawing to detect items such as shading, frowning mouth, erasures, etc. One point was given for each item that met the criteria outlined in the manual. For instance, a baseline was scored if the child drew a ground line, grass, etc. The manual included detailed descriptions of the criteria considered.

SOURCE OF ITEMS:

Item development contained an exhaustive review of the literature on indicators of emotional disturbance. Additionally, items were considered indicators if they occurred infrequently in normal populations and showed appropriate psychometric properties. Items were initially categorized by figure size, placement on the page, stance, integrations, omissions, shading, etc. Independent raters were used to review the items, modify them, and eliminate ambiguities in the scoring system. Following a pilot study, the authors found that the DAP: SPED had good interrater and intrarater reliability. Also, it was an effective device for discriminating normal from emotionally disturbed populations.

VALIDITY AS DETERMINED BY THE AUTHORS:

The discriminant validity of the DAP: SPED was examined with a group of 81 students placed in a special educational setting matched to

81 normal students from the standardization sample. Every special education student was diagnosed as having a severe behavioral handicapped which included children with learning disabilities and emotional problems. The DAP: SPED significantly discriminated between the two groups.

Another study examined 49 adolescents (16 females and 33 males) attending a psychiatric residential treatment facility for the seriously emotionally disturbed. More than 85 percent of the sample was labeled as conduct disordered. The sample was matched to the standardization sample based on age, gender, race, and geographic region. All students were administered the DAP: SPED in a group setting. Again, the authors found that the assessment significantly discriminated between the two groups in that the residential students earned higher scores.

A third study involved 58 children and adolescents (8 females and 50 males) in special education placements. This sample was predominantly white. The sample was matched according to age, gender, race, and geographic region. The special education group earned significantly higher scores on the DAP: SPED than the standard group. The results again demonstrated the discriminant validity of the DAP: SPED.

In a fourth study, 54 children and adolescents attending a day treatment facility for the emotionally disturbed were matched to the standardization sample. Naglieri and Pfeiffer (1992) found that the day treatment individuals earned significantly higher scores on the DAP: SPED than the standardization sample. "The present findings, therefore, suggest that the DAP: SPED system, because of its objective and uniform scoring rules, nationally representative standardization sample, and good reliability, may be relatively more useful for evaluating human figure drawings and may be shown to hold promise as a screening test" (Naglieri & Pfeiffer, 1992, p. 158).

Although some human figure drawing tests have been used as indicators of intelligence, the authors sought to prove that the DAP: SPED was unrelated to intellectual functioning. Using the MAT–SF (Matrix Anologies Test—Short Form) test (Naglieri, 1985) scores of the standardization sample, the authors found that very low, nonsignificant correlations with the DAP: SPED. The MAT–SF test, a nonverbal test, used the progressive matrix format to measure intelligence.

The authors examined the standardization sample for cultural differences. Nonsignificant differences were found between black and white students. Additionally, no differences were found between Hispanic and non-Hispanic students. "These findings, like the analyses of race differences, however should be considered tentative until additional investigations are conducted" (Naglieri et al., 1991, p. 20).

RELIABILITY AS DETERMINED BY THE AUTHORS:

Using the scores obtained from the standardization sample, the authors provided internal consistency and standard errors of measurement for each age group. They found that the DAP: SPED had an appropriate level of internal reliability for screening purposes (range of .67 to .78).

An earlier scoring system was used to determine interrater and intrarater reliability data. Twenty-five drawings were scored two times by the same rater, and then the drawings were scored by different raters. The qualifications of the raters were not discussed. Interrater reliability was reported to be .91 and intrarater reliability was reported to be .94. Another study examined the interrater reliability of the DAP: SPED. Interrater reliability was reported to be .84 and intrarater reliability, using a one month interval, was reported to be .83.

A sample of 67 students attending a school for learning problems (learning disabilities, emotional, behavioral problems, and brain injury) were used to examine the stability of the DAP: SPED. Other demographic characteristics of the sample were not discussed. Using a one week interval, no significant differences in scores were found, providing some support for the stability of the DAP: SPED.

RESEARCH USING THE DAP:

Over the years, there has been much controversy concerning the validity and reliability of human figure drawing tests. Motta and colleagues (1993) reviewed the DAP: SPED. They asked: "Why anyone would use figure drawings to identify such an obviously disturbed group when simple behavioral observation would suffice, is left to the reader's imagination" (Motta et al., 1993, p. 165). They reported that Naglieri and Pfeiffer's (1992) study identified less than half of the psychiatrically disturbed group. In other words, 48.15 percent of the clinical sample was identified as in need of further evaluation. Since the majority of the sample was not identified, the authors criticized the accuracy rate of the scoring procedure. "These sad data speak for themselves" (Motta et al., 1993, p. 165).

Naglieri (1993) responded to these authors by stating that Motta et al. (1993) "have missed the point that DAP: SPED offers a significant improvement in the use of the draw a person technique as a means of evaluating the presence of emotional problems" (p. 171). Further, Naglieri argued that simple behavioral observations were not sufficient to correctly classify students. In support of Naglieri (1993), Bardos (1993) contended that Motta, et al. (1993) neglected to comment on the extensive and representative standardization sample used in the DAP: SPED. Additionally, Bardos (1993) commented that it was valid to investigate previously labeled, emotionally disturbed children. This was done to provide discriminant validity evidence. "Could it be possible that some of them find it impossible or extremely difficult to conduct a behavioral assessment for every student in their system as the authors recommend" (Bardos, 1993, p. 180)?

The remainder of the research conducted to date was on the DAP: QSS. Since the DAP: SPED stated that the drawings obtained can be used to determine cognitive functions, research on the DAP: QSS will be briefly reviewed. Neisworth and Butler (1990) wrote a test review on the DAP: QSS. They stated that the manual was comprehensive, clear, and concise. Administration and interpretation guidelines were well outlined. "The inclusion of the self-instruction competency test is an excellent way to learn how to administer the DAP and to be assured that when one is scoring the test, the best possible results will be obtained" (Neisworth & Butler, 1990, p. 190). The scoring system covered detail, proportion, and parts of the body. As with the DAP: SPED, raw scores were converted to standard scores. The manual used the same normative sample as the DAP: SPED. Test-retest reliability ranged from .60 to .89 for the total score and from .58 to .70 for individual scores. Interrater reliability was reported to be .86 to .95. Intrarater reliability ranged from .89 to .98. Construct validity was provided in that children's scores increased with age. Concurrent validity evidence was provided by comparing the assessment to the Goodenough-Harris scoring system (r = .77). Since the DAP correlated higher with the MAT–SF than with the MAS math and reading, the reviewers concluded that the DAP was measuring something other than achievement. Other studies found no scoring differences across race or gender. Although the reviewers found the DAP: QSS an improvement over other assessments, they stated that "construct validity is arguable and treatment utility is questionable" (Neisworth & Butler, 1990, p. 194).

Kamphause and Pleiss (1991) reached a similar conclusion when reviewing the DAP: QSS. "While the DAP is the best drawing technique available, its concurrent validly evidence does not support the use of such instruments as measures on intelligence" (p. 395). The authors stressed that the DAP: QSS was not a valid nor reliable measure of intelligence or a screener for intelligence. Motta and colleagues (1993) agreed that the DAP: QSS offered little evidence in support of concurrent and predictive validity. For additional information on the DAP: QSS, please refer to the following authors (Naglieri, 1988; Prewett et al., 1989; & Wisniewski & Naglieri, 1989)

DESIRABLE FEATURES:

The DAP: SPED manual was clear and concise. Administration and scoring guidelines were clearly outlined. The assessment required little time for administration. The templates were helpful when scoring the drawings. Case examples were clearly structured and demonstrated the scoring system adequately.

UNDESIRABLE FEATURES:

The fact that the directions read "I would like you to draw for me" may promote transference issues with the examiner if the child already has a pretesting relationship. If the directions were changed to read "Draw a picture . . . ," it would avoid any extraneous influences on the drawing itself. There was a performance demand in the way the directions read. Since the child has only five minutes to complete the drawing, this may prove to be very frustrating. Also, to make the best picture you can, a child may need more than five minutes. It was not clear from the instructions if the child was aware that she only has five minutes to complete the drawing. If children are not aware, they may become upset and have difficulty completing the assessment.

OVERALL EVALUATION:

The test designers provided an excellent standardization sample that outlined demographic characteristics clearly and completely. The manual was easy to read. Instructions for administration, scoring, and interpretation were very detailed, yet clear.

Construct validity evidence was weak. This was a general complaint about most human figure drawing tests. Discriminant validity evidence was moderate to strong. The DAP: SPED appeared to discriminate between normal populations and special populations. One criticism was that the special populations included a number of individuals, some with learning disabilities others with emotional problems. Since not all children with learning disabilities, such as dyslexia, have emotional problems, additional research is needed to determine exactly what the DAP: SPED is screening.

Reliability evidence appeared strong. No significant differences were found after a one week interval, indicating the stability of the instrument. Future studies may vary the length of this interval provided that it does not exceed six months (Anastasi, 1988). The authors could have provided more information on the qualifications of the raters. It was not clear if the test designers also served as raters in the studies cited.

Although the manual stated that the drawings could be used as measures of intellectual functioning, there was no evidence provided. The manual refers the reader to the DAP: QSS manual for scoring information. It appeared from the research conducted to date that the DAP cannot be used as a measure of intellectual functioning since predictive and concurrent validity evidence was lacking.

REFERENCES

Anastasi, A. (1988). *Psychological testing.* 6th ed. New York: Macmillan.

Bardos, A.N. (1993). Human figure drawings: Abusing the abused. *School Psychology Quarterly, 8(3),* 177–181.

Kamphause, R.W., and Pleiss, K.L. (1991). Draw-a-Person techniques: Tests in search of a construct. *Journal of School Psychology, 29,* 395–401.

Motta, R.W., Little, S.G., and Tobin, M.I. (1993). The use and abuse of human figure drawings. *School Psychology Quarterly, 8(3),* 162–169.

Naglieri, J.A. (1985). *Matrix Analogies Test—Short Form.* New York: Psychological Corporation.

Naglieri, J.A. (1988). *Draw a Person: A quantitative scoring system.* New York: Psychological Corporation.

Naglieri, J.A. (1993). Human figure drawings in perspective. *School Psychology Quarterly, 8(3),* 170–176.

Naglieri, J.A., McNeish, T.J., and Bardos, A.N. (1991). *Draw a Person: Screening Procedure for Emotional Disturbance.* Austin, TX: Pro-Ed.

Naglieri, J.A., and Pfeiffer, S.I. (1992). Performance of disruptive behavior disordered and normal samples on the Draw a Person: Screening Procedure for Emotional Disturbance. *Psychological Assessment, 4(2),* 156–159.

Neisworth, J.T., and Butler, R.J. (1990). Test review: Draw a Person: A quantitative scoring system. *Journal of Psychoeducational Assessment, 8,* 190–194.

Prewett, P.N., Bardos, A.N., and Naglieri, J.A. (1989). Assessment of mentally retarded children with the Matrix Analogies Test-Short Form, Draw a Person: A Quantitative Scoring System, and the Kaufman Test of Education Achievement. *Psychology in the Schools, 26,* p. 254–260.

Wisniewski, J.J., and Naglieri, J.A. (1989). Validity of the Draw a Person: A quantitative scoring system with the WISC–R. *Journal of Psychoeducational Assessment, 7,* 346–351.

Chapter 11

MAGAZINE PHOTO COLLAGE

TITLE:	Magazine Photo Collage (MPC)
AGE:	age limit not presented
YEAR:	1993
PURPOSE:	designed to reveal client's conflicts, defense mechanisms, and styles of functioning; interpretation based on the client's procedural approach to the task, pictorial content, and free associations
SCORES:	based on guidelines for interpretation
MANUAL:	manual (183 pages); illustrations (93 pages); profile (21 pages); reliability data (none reported); validity data (none reported)
TIME LIMIT:	to be completed in one session (time limit not otherwise defined)
COST:	$23.95–$28.95 for testing manual
AUTHOR:	Landgarten, Helen B
PUBLISHER:	Brunner/Mazel, Inc., 19 Union Square, New York, NY, 10003.

INTRODUCTION:

The Magazine Photo Collage (MPC) was designed for multicultural assessment and treatment. Rather than using a standardized test, such as the Thematic Apperception Test (TAT) that represents only one race, the MPC may be standardized by the therapist to fit specialized populations. Depending on the therapist's population of interest and expertise, she may provide images varying in age, gender, and race. As with the TAT (Murray, 1943), the focus of the MPC was on content. Unlike other projective assessments, the materials used for administration may vary from one therapist to the next. The box of photo images continuously changes. As a result, the MPC was an empowering process:

> Because clients choose their own collage images, they are provided with a rich symbolic vocabulary for self-expression, and one that is individualized to suit their own needs. The opportunity to exercise some control over the selection

process can lessen inhibitions and resistant factors for many clients. This facet also encourages the positive transference and hastens the establishment of a therapeutic alliance. (Landgarten, 1993, p. 2)

Completed collages allowed the therapist to confront the meaning of the images, make an intervention, offer an interpretation, or simply note the content before going on to the next phase of the assessment.

Since 1967, Landgarten has been addressing the problems of cross-cultural counseling. Monocultural assumptions of mental health, derogatory stereotypes of minorities, and limited knowledge of cultural groups result in inappropriate and ineffective counseling approaches (Sue & Sue, 1990). Additionally, cultural values, class values, and language variables also limit counseling effectiveness. By trying to select images that match the client's culture, Landgarten (1993) hoped to resolve some of the problems of cross cultural counseling. As a result, she found that therapy progressed at a faster pace. This in turn, fostered positive transference and a stronger relationship with her clients. In her book on the MPC, Landgarten (1993) presented case examples of Asian, African, Hispanic, and Caucasian clients' work on several types of issues: School phobia, anorexia nervosa, loss, suicidal ideation, and posttraumatic stress disorder, to name a few. The MPC also had the capability of addressing individuals who come from two or more racial groups. This was particularly valuable when dealing with racial identity issues.

PURPOSE AND RECOMMENDED USE:

The MPC was designed to generate information about client conflicts, defense mechanisms, and styles of functioning (Landgarten, 1993). It may be used with any cultural group, provided that the therapist can include photos that relate to the client's cultural background. Also, it may be incorporated into the treatment process by including tasks that have a thematic orientation or offer free choice. "Regardless of the way in which the clinician proceeds, the client's collage becomes the document that gains access to conscious as well as unconscious material" (Landgarten, 1993, p. 3). Age limit and the possibility of group administration were not discussed.

DIMENSIONS THAT THE TEST
PURPORTS TO MEASURE:

The First Task of the MPC involved a free choice collage of miscellaneous images. According to Landgarten (1993), this task will convey information on how the collage was constructed. For instance, the therapist may note how the images were handled, glued, and placed on the page. Additionally, the counselor may observe the document for specific messages or themes.

Involving a collage of people images, the Second Task was said to indicate the client's perception of trust within herself, significant others, or the therapist. It explored the connection between action and cognition by writing what each image was thinking and saying. This facet of the task may reveal congruencies and disparities. The Second Task was a measure of the client's self-image and generated information about the transference relationship. How this task indicated transference was unclear.

For the Third Task, the client was asked to pick out pictures of people or miscellaneous items that stand for something good and something bad. This task revealed images that the client associated with positive feelings and negative emotions. The therapist may consider the use of only people images, only miscellaneous images, or a combination of the two groups. Landgarten (1993) purported that the use of humorous images and miscellaneous images was a distancing mechanism.

In the Fourth Task, the client was presented with a restriction: Selecting only one picture from the people box. This task measured the person's positive or negative outlook on life. "This will illuminate the individual's attitude, coping mechanisms, and whether or not problem-solving through alternatives is part of his/her life-style" (Landgarten, 1993, p. 11). Since Landgarten (1993) did not expand further on this statement, the exact nature of determining the client's attitude remained unclear.

ADMINISTRATION:

Landgarten (1993) recommended that all four MPC tasks be completed in one session (length of session was not discussed), beginning with Task One and ending with Task Four. It was the administrator's choice whether or not to set a time limit. If one was set, then the therapist should consider pressure factors when doing the assessment. Qualifications of the administrator were not discussed.

Collages were completed on newsprint or white paper, 16 by 20 inches. After the assessment phase, the therapist had the option of using colored construction paper. The following tools were required: A thin black marker, medium black marker, ball point pen, round tip scissors, and a lead pencil. In order to observe handling, Landgarten (1993) stressed that liquid glue should be used during the assessment. After the assessment phase was complete, the client may use a glue stick. Overall, Landgarten (1993) was very clear in the types of materials required and the manner in which the MPC may be administered.

NORM GROUPS:

The MPC was not standardized on a population. It included case examples representing various cultural groups. The manner in which these cases were selected was unclear. Although the cases denoted various cultural groups and both genders, very few children were included. It may be that Landgarten (1993) felt that the MPC was more appropriate for adolescents and adult populations.

INTERPRETATION OF SCORES:

The assessment process was divided into three parts: process, content, and free associations. Landgarten (1993) endorsed an analytical approach in that each process must be viewed separately as opposed to the whole. In the first part of the assessment, the therapist viewed how the client approached the task. Landgarten (1993) outlined seven components of this process. One component was the way that the client looked through the box of pictures. Landgarten (1993) expressed that the demeanor may be categorized as follows: lackadaisical, serious, casual, disdainful, angry, anxious, and so forth. Additionally, she maintained that clients who were extremely cautious in any of the categories may have one or more of the following problems: passivity, depression, ambivalence, inability to deal with emotion, problems with decision making, or obsessive-compulsive characteristics. Also, clients who recklessly completed the collage and had problems with boundaries may have serious psychopathology such as bipolar depression, borderline personality disorder, drug addiction, or psychosis. According to Landgarten (1993), functioning individuals will look through many images, take a reasonable amount of time, use appropriate glue, and have some white space surrounding their images. She then furnished examples that illustrated the first part of the assessment process.

The second part of the MPC concerned evaluation of the pictorial content. The therapist observed inclusions and exclusions. For the people pictures, Landgarten (1993) designed a list of eight questions. For example, "Are all the photographs either of men or women, or boys or girls" (p. 20)? The client's free associations were taken into account. Projections about self, significant others, and transference issues were considered. According to Landgarten (1993), the Miscellaneous images "may disclose the person's value system, attitude toward life, concerns, fears, wishes" (Landgarten, 1993, p. 20). Also, the images may reveal the client's developmental level. Images that should alert the therapist included a loped rope, crashed cars, wrecked homes, broken glass, weapons, or pills.

The third part of the assessment involved free associations. Any verbal response was acceptable. Landgarten (1993) claimed that the client's verbal associations were critical to validate the therapists hypotheses about the client.

SOURCE OF ITEMS:

The MPC consisted of black and white and color magazine images that were culturally homogeneous to the client's population. These images were selected by the counselor and divided into two categories: People and Miscellaneous Items. Printed words were removed from the images. In addition, the images were NOT carefully cut in order to provide more information about the manner in which the client completed the collage. The images for the People box comprised some of the following: people from different cultures, reality oriented (avoiding glamorous images), showing movement as well as static positions, and included different environments. Males and females of various ages and facial expressions were included. Miscellaneous items generally came from ads and encompassed a variety of inanimate objects such as trucks, jewelry, tools, furniture, and houses.

How Landgarten (1993) selected these four particular tasks was unclear. If the tasks had a theoretical foundation in art therapy or psychotherapy, it was not presented in the manual. Additional information was needed on the historical development of the tasks.

VALIDITY AND RELIABILITY AS DETERMINED BY THE AUTHOR:

Landgarten (1993) openly admitted that she did not investigate the reliability or validity of this instrument.

> Suggestions or interpretations are based on my many years of clinical practice. This book does not lay claim to the exact meanings for particular images. In fact, images can represent different meanings to different clients. (Landgarten, 1993, p. 2)

Establishing reliability evidence for the MPC may be possible. Landgarten's assessment factors can be incorporated into a scoring sheet used to rate the client's demeanor as well as the pictorial content. Interrater reliability can be checked in this manner. Since the historical development and theoretical background of the MPC was not discussed, it was difficult to project a possible study of validity.

RESEARCH USING THE MPC:

To date, there was no research on the MPC. Instead, the literature contained a few articles on the use of collage in general. For instance, Katz (1987) used photo collage as a treatment modality for working with a group of eight-year-old females.

> the affective and cognitive arenas of the preconscious are allowed to surface, with one's picture providing a safe distance for looking at one's self. The inspiration which one feels at this moment combines spontaneous ideas, visions, social and personal desires, all of which describe the individual. (Katz, 1987, p. 83)

Katz (1987) asserted that through photo collage, clients were able to cultivate an empathic connections with others, ventilate personal concerns, and master skills and aesthetic development. In working with young girls, Katz (1987) found that ego functions were strengthened. Frustration tolerance increased and impulsiveness decreased. The purpose of her work was to foster conflict resolution skills. "This issue of identity, in relation to one's individuation and the struggle toward more mature realization of one's unique potentials, is a major theme explored through this modality, and highly congruent with the purposes of social group work" (Katz, 1987, p. 89). The changes in the group were observed by the researcher and were not in relation to measured changes in demeanor.

Another article focused on a secondary school teacher's use of photo collage in her classroom. Jones (1990) instructed her students to trace a silhouette of a partner's face. Students then pasted images into their own silhouette. Next, they worked on the space around the silhouette. In the surrounding area, some students represented one of the four elements others created symbols of their Zodiac sign. Overall, Jones (1990) found that this activity was very pleasurable for the students.

Reissman (1992) used collage work with students to increase multi-cultural awareness. By breaking the students into groups, she had them look for one particular racial group in the daily newspapers. They were asked to make predictions about how many news items would be devoted to the ethnic group and what section of the newspaper would contain stories about the group. Collages were created out of the articles found in the papers. "These students found that through selection of images, the news media could perpetuate, create, or defuse stereotypes" (Reissman, 1992, p. 52).

Although these articles were interesting, they represented only a qualitative approach to collage work. It would be interesting to see empirical studies that evaluated the effectiveness of collages, specifically the MPC, by examining self-esteem, social reticence, or depression. This information would strengthen the rationale of photo collage work in general as well as the use of the MPC as a therapeutic assessment.

DESIRABLE FEATURES:

The MPC process was empowering because the client had control over the selection of magazine images. Landgarten (1993) designed a four-task assessment protocol which was simple to administer and fit into the treatment process easily. It avoided the cookbook approach to art therapy assessment in that interpretation was primarily based on the client's free associations and the therapist's observation of the manner in which the collage was completed. Collage work was less threatening for some clients who may feel intimidated when drawing, painting, or sculpting. Landgarten (1993) presented clear guidelines for the administration of the MPC, materials needed, and case examples that illustrated the interpretation of the assessment. Also, the MPC appeared to counter some of the problems inherent in cross-cultural counseling by taking into consideration images familiar to clients with diverse backgrounds.

UNDESIRABLE FEATURES:

The assessment used only images of people and inanimate objects. This limited the scope of the assessment in that animal and nature images were not included. In my experience, animal images were often used in collages and drawings. Clients seemed to identify with them. Important information may be neglected if the client was not able to select nature images or images of animals.

The fact that the MPC was to be completed in one session was confining. The time period for a session may vary from one therapist to the next. When following Landgarten's (1993) guidelines and using a 50-minute time limit, I found that clients were rushing through the assessment in order to complete the four tasks. Naturally, this interfered with the interpretation of the assessment. I varied Landgarten's (1993) approach by allowing the client to take as much time as needed to complete the MPC. Another weakness of the MPC was that the tasks were viewed separately. With an assessment of this nature, common themes among the tasks should be considered.

Interpretation of the tasks may be difficult. The exact nature of how the collage measured transference and counter transference issues was unclear. The same holds true for the interpretation of the client's attitude from one particular image. Additional information was needed on the interpretation of the collage tasks.

OVERALL EVALUATION:

Since Landgarten has been working with collages for over thirty years, it would have been helpful to include information on the historical development of the MPC. Also, it would have been interesting to learn how these four tasks were selected to comprise the MPC. A reference list including other people's work with collages would be practical. Further, a list of other possible collage tasks to guide therapy would have been useful to ongoing treatment.

The lack of validity and reliability information was regretful, but it is not impossible to obtain. A scoring guide can be constructed to record information on the assessment. This would be beneficial in the collection of interrater reliability evidence. Another interesting study that would have promoted validity would be to examine the variation in time when completing the MPC: a single session versus as many sessions as the client requires. Since Landgarten (1993) claimed that the MPC was a multicultural assessment, research should be completed to sanction this point.

The use of the case method appeared to be the approach of choice with this art therapy assessment. Although the case method fosters insight on the use of art therapy, it has several limitations. First, case studies are not representative samples. Additionally, the observers are not blind and therefore, may not be objective. Lastly, the case method does not utilize a comparison group. These are important considerations when reviewing any type of assessment.

Overall, the MPC portended to be an empowering approach when working with clients. It offered the client a choice in image selection and interpretation of the collage. Additionally, it reduced the possibility of cultural bias by including images consistent with a client's cultural background. I have attempted to promote client autonomy and responsibility by requiring people to contribute images to the collection. Also, I have encouraged the use of animal, tree, and water images. The MPC may increase a client's awareness of self by yielding information about inner conflicts and relationships with others.

REFERENCES

Jones, L. (1990). In your element: Students often "fill their heads" with all kinds of ideas. *School Arts, January*, 36–37.

Katz, S.L. (1987). Photocollage as a therapeutic modality for working with groups. *Social Work with Groups, 10(4)*, 83–89.

Landgarten, H.B. (1993). *Magazine Photo Collage*. New York, NY: Brunner Mazel.

Murray, H.A. (1943). *Thematic Apperception Test*. Cambridge, MA: Harvard University Press.

Reissman, R. (1992). Multicultural awareness collages. *Educational Leadership, December–January*, 51–52.

Sue, D.W. and Sue, D. (1990). *Counseling the culturally different*. New York: John Wiley & Sons.

Chapter 12

BELIEF ART THERAPY ASSESSMENT

TITLE: Belief Art Therapy Assessment (BATA)
AGE: age limit not presented
YEAR: 1994
PURPOSE: designed to understand the spiritual dimensions of a client; interpretation based on the client's developmental level, subject matter, formal qualities of artwork, and client attitude
SCORES: based on interpretation guidelines
MANUAL: manual (169 pages); illustrations (34 pages); profile (26 pages); reliability data (none reported); validity data (none reported)
TIME LIMIT: no time limit for administration
COST: $42.00 for testing manual ($29.95 for paperback)
AUTHOR: Horovitz-Darby, Ellen G.
PUBLISHER: Charles C Thomas Publisher, 2600 South First Street, Springfield, IL 62794-9265.

INTRODUCTION:

The Belief Art Therapy Assessment (BATA: Horovitz-Darby, 1994) emanated from the exploration of mourning and loss issues. "Beginning with these losses reconnects the patient to his very origin of dis-ease (e.g. symptomatic discomfort) and sets the stage for inclusion of the spiritual dimension" (Horovitz-Darby, 1994, p. 14). While many professionals in the field have equated the pursuit of religion with poor mental health, Horovitz-Darby (1994) professed that investigating spirituality was motivated by a search for meaning in one's life. This sense of purpose served to connect the client to society or community. She endorsed McNiff's (1992) concept of art as healing, a mystical experience that fostered integration. As McNiff (1992), she confronted client pain and suffering as a method of moving the client toward growth.

Since the field of art therapy was just beginning to explore spirituality, Horovitz-Darby (1994) developed the BATA. This assessment was fashioned to explore the client's belief systems as it related to personal and familial functioning.

> In fact, I ardently maintain that families can be instructed how to care for themselves within a brief time frame. The argument stems from the fact that they have been caring for themselves all along, even when doing it badly. All the more reason to tap into a client's belief system; for in doing so, the therapist can empower the identified patient yet align with the hierarchical powers. (Horovitz-Darby, 1994, p. 28)

As Ellison (1991), Horovitz-Darby perceived that religious beliefs may affect the client's coping skills and ability to deal with stress. Additionally, exploration of religious symbols and beliefs may provide an avenue through which the client can understand and integrate life experiences. Corsini and Wedding (1989) defined religion as the "expression of an archetypal need to endow our human existence with meaning" (p. 140). As Horovitz-Darby (1994), they alleged that analyzing religious imagery may help the client contend with his inner resources and serve to empower her.

PURPOSE AND RECOMMENDED USE:

Horovitz-Darby (1994) recommended that the BATA be used only when the client had questions about his/her spirituality. Horovitz-Darby (1994) warned that for clients who are emotionally disturbed or psychotic, the BATA may not be appropriate in that it may exacerbate their condition. The BATA began with an interview intended to gather information on the client's past and present religious beliefs. Next, the client was given two directives and asked to make art products in response to each. Since Horovitz-Darby (1994) had difficulty conducting the BATA in public school settings, it may not be appropriate for school psychologists to administer this assessment. From reading the manual, it appeared that the BATA can be used by private practitioners in the event that a client expresses a need to explore spiritual dimensions. It may be used with religious individuals as well as agnostics or atheists. The BATA may be utilized to elicit information on client issues as well as determine the course of treatment.

DIMENSIONS THAT THE TEST PURPORTS TO MEASURE:

The BATA was created to provide an indication of a client's spiritual belief system. The assessment consisted of two directives. The first directive was stated as follows:

> Have you ever thought about how the universe was created and who or what was responsible for our creation? Many people have a belief in God; if you also have a belief in God, would you draw, paint, or sculpt what God means to you. (Horovitz-Darby, 1994, p. 32)

For people who did not believe in God, the administrator may ask what beliefs the client supports. Should the client state that he believes in nothing, the administrator may request that the client represent that using art media. After the first directive, the client was given a post-assessment interrogation. These questions attempted to ascertain what the client made and what it meant to her. The second directive was stipulated as follows:

> Some people believe that there is an opposite of God. If you believe there is an opposite force, could you also draw, paint or sculpt the meaning of that? (Horovitz-Darby, 1994, p. 33)

Next, the postassessment interrogation was administered again.

ADMINISTRATION:

Horovitz-Darby (1994) enumerated a series of media that may be used for the BATA. The list included two-dimensional drafting media, two-dimensional painting media, three-dimensional media, and types of paper. This was one of the few assessments that offered a wide variety of media. The administrator conducted the interview first. Since clinicians vary in their skills as interviewers, Horovitz-Darby (1994) furnished some general questions for the query. She offered the administrator the option of adding or deleting questions depending on the client's personality and psychological parameters. Next, the client was given the first directive followed by a post-assessment interrogation. The BATA concluded with the second directive followed by another postassessment interrogation. The qualifications of the administrator were not discussed.

NORM GROUPS:

The BATA was not standardized on a population. Instead, the manual contained a series of case examples that comprised members of the clergy; adult artists; emotionally disturbed children and adolescents; and a suicidal, bulimic anorectic. The case examples were thorough compared to some authors (Burns & Kaufman, 1972; Burns, 1987) who only provided minimal information on the client background. Horovitz-Darby (1994) depicted genograms and photographs in the case examples.

INTERPRETATION OF SCORES:

Interpretation of the BATA was based on developmental level, formal qualities of the artwork, subject matter, and client attitude. Development was determined by Lowenfeld and Brittain's (1987) stages of cognitive development. Horovitz-Darby (1994) outlined a series of parameters to guide the reader in the interpretation of the art products. For instance, formal qualities of the artwork considered the creation or lack of creating a product. If a client was unable to produce a product, it may indicate withdrawal, playful experimentation, destructive behavior, extreme duress or anxiety due to nature of the topic, or resistance (Horovitz-Darby, 1994). Subject matter deliberated common themes and blatant contradictions. Attitude was the client's demeanor as the product was created. Response to specific media, avoidance of materials, gratification, and self-perceptions were other considerations relating to client attitude.

Horovitz-Darby (1994) cited a model invented by Fowler (1981) that was used in the interpretation of the BATA. Fowler (1981) constructed a stage theory for spiritual development, similar to Kohlberg's (1981) theory of moral development. This six stage theory was clearly outlined in Horovitz-Darby's work.

SOURCE OF ITEMS:

The creation of the BATA originated from Horovitz-Darby's (1994) "conviction that people's belief systems were indigenous to their operational and systems functioning" (p. 28). Looking back on the work of Coles (1990), who asked children to draw a picture of God, Horovitz-Darby (1994) decided that some religious factions might take offense to this request. She redesigned Coles' (1990) directive to provide an indication of the "meaning" of God as opposed to the representation of God. Additionally, she expanded Coles' (1990) two-dimensional drawing request to include a myriad of two- and three-dimensional art media.

VALIDITY AND RELIABILITY AS DETERMINED BY THE AUTHOR:

Horovitz-Darby (1994) did not investigate the validity or reliability of the BATA. Since it was a recently developed assessment, there was no research to date that examined the BATA. "Although the data could be analyzed, categorized, and converted into mathematical computation, my precise desire was to create a battery that recognized the spiritual dimension of a person and contributed pertinent information in order to effect treatment" (Horovitz-Darby, 1994, p. 27).

DESIRABLE FEATURES:

The BATA offered a free choice of art media. Given that some clients may be anxious about exploring spiritual issues, this was a valuable improvement over other art therapy assessments that were limited to using only pencil drawings. Also, the BATA can be used with agnostics or atheists. Horovitz-Darby (1994) supplied a list of questions and suggestions when working with these individuals. The manual was very descriptive and included several case examples that demonstrated the use of the BATA.

UNDESIRABLE FEATURES:

A form for recording the interview, postassessment interrogations, formal qualities of the artwork, and client attitude would have been helpful. Creating a checklist may be a first step in furnishing reliability information for the BATA. Since examiner qualifications were not discussed, guidelines for interpretation could have been more detailed. Individuals with little clinical experience or training in art therapy may find the BATA difficult to interpret.

OVERALL EVALUATION:

Horovitz-Darby included several case examples in the manual. Although she described Fowler's (1981) theory of spiritual development in detail, she did not address its application in several of the case examples. This may be the key to providing validity evidence for the BATA. Creating a checklist that outlined spiritual development (Fowler, 1981), cognitive development (Lowenfeld and Brittain, 1987), and qualitative interpretations of the artwork (Horovitz-Darby, 1994) may serve as the foundation for providing both reliability and validity evidence. Additionally, Horovitz-Darby (1988) created the Cognitive Art Therapy Assessment (CATA) in which she clearly detailed the interpretation of paint, clay, and drawing media. Incorporating these guidelines for interpretation would have been worthwhile when interpreting the BATA. Additional information on the reliability and validity of the BATA was needed.

To date, the BATA was the only assessment in art therapy that explored a client's spiritual development. Since spirituality was an important facet of many people's life, this assessment was long overdue. Additionally, the client was offered a wide variety of media in order to complete the assessment. Most art therapy tests were limited to pencil drawings. Another important feature of this assessment was that it can be used with atheists or agnostics; it was not restricted to individuals who subscribe to the traditional religions. Although the BATA may not be appropriate for all clients, it did offer an option to those individuals who were ready to explore their spiritual nature.

REFERENCES

Burns, R.C. (1987). *Kinetic-House-Tree-Person-Drawings: An interpretive manual.* New York, NY: Brunner/Mazel.

Burns, R.C., and Kaufman, S.H. (1972). *Actions, styles, and symbols in Kinetic Family Drawings (K–F–D): An interpretive manual.* New York: Brunner/Mazel.

Coles, R. (1990). *The spiritual life of children.* Boston, MA: Houghton-Mifflin.

Corsini, R.J. and Wedding, D. (1989). *Current psychotherapies.* Itasca, IL: F.E. Peacock.

Ellison, C.G. (1991). Religious involvement and subjective well-being. *Journal of Health and Social Behavior, 32(1),* 80–99.

Fowler, J.W. (1981). *Stages of faith: The psychology of human development and the quest for meaning.* San Francisco, CA: Harper.

Horovitz-Darby, E.G. (1988). Art therapy assessment of a minimally language skilled deaf child. Chapter 11 in *Mental health assessment of deaf clients: Special conditions.*

Proceedings from the 1988 University of California's Center on Deafness Conference, ADARA, 115–127.

Horovitz-Darby, E.G. (1994). *Spiritual art therapy: An alternate path.* Springfield, IL: Charles C Thomas.

Kohlberg, L. (1981). *The philosophy of moral development.* New York: Harper & Row.

Lowenfeld, V., and Brittain, W.L. (1987). *Creative and mental growth.* 8th ed. New York: Macmillan.

McNiff, S. (1992). *Art as medicine: Creating a therapy of the imagination.* Boston, MA: Shambhala.

Chapter 13

RECOMMENDATIONS

Considering the findings in the previous chapters of this book, this section will summarize the strengths and weaknesses of the art therapy assessments reviewed. Recommendations will be made based on the assessment's reliability and validity evidence as well as the desirable and undesirable features. Additionally, the clinical usefulness of the assessment will be evaluated based upon research to date and my clinical experience.

HUMAN FIGURE DRAWING TEST (1968):

Koppitz (1968) conducted thorough research to provide evidence for the usefulness of the HFD. She clearly described developmental items and emotional indicators of human figure drawings by utilizing case studies. Mental development, school achievement, organic conditions, and personality characteristics were a few of the areas reviewed using human figure drawings. Unfortunately, interpretations of the HFDs were based on these case studies. Additionally, quantitative scoring procedures were not demonstrated in the case examples.

Koppitz's (1968) HFD did show some discriminant validity, particularly with high achievers compared to low achievers. Although she demonstrated that the HFD can discriminate between shy and aggressive children, other researchers were unable to produce the same results (Lingren, 1971; Norford & Barakat, 1990). Discriminant validity for the HFD was lacking: The HFD did not discriminate sexually abused, learning disabled, or aggressive children from well adjusted populations. This author agrees with Motta et al. (1993) who argued that the HFD was not a reliable or valid instrument for assessing intelligence. Information on the reliability of the HFD needs to be examined. Since the standardization sample was selected over 30 years ago, future research should focus on reestablishing norms for the HFD. Clinicians may use the HFD in conjunction with other assessments in order to provide information on client issues. In my work with sexual abuse survivors, omission of body parts was a common feature of HFDs. Additionally, sexual abuse survivors typically only draw the head and neglect the lower part of the body. This assessment does require clinical experience when interpreting drawings. It is recommended that the HFD not be used as a measure of intelligence; rather, as a tool to illuminate client concerns and self-perceptions.

KINETIC FAMILY DRAWINGS (1972):

Burns and Kaufman (1972) added a kinetic component to traditional family drawings to create the KFD. This assessment provided an indication of a person's familial relationships and issues. The case examples were helpful in understanding how the authors intended the KFD to be used. Overall, the KFD potentially yielded valuable information about familial relationships as well as self-concept. The authors created a grid to quantify information about the KFD; yet, they did not present guidelines for the interpretation of measurements.

There was very little information on how the test was developed. Additionally, no information was given on who was able to administer the KFD and their qualifications. Interpretation may be difficult, given the ambiguity in the test terms and lack of examples for the grid information. Objective scoring systems have been developed for the KFD (Cummings, 1980; Mostkoff & Lazarus, 1983). With training, interrater reliability has been established (McPhee & Wegner, 1976). Test-retest reliability evidence was weak, suggesting that the KFD may be sensitive to mood changes. Validity evidence was also mixed. Studies that examined the KFD as a possible screening device had mixed results. Research indicated that cultural differences as well as sex differences were found when using the KFD (Cabacungan, 1985). Generally, the exact nature of what the KFD measures was not clear.

Despite these limitations, the KFD showed promise as a tool that yielded information about a child's personality state. Research indicated that the KFD was a particularly useful instrument when evaluating children who were suspected sexual abuse survivors. Further evidence was needed to determine whether or not the KFD can adequately distinguish between other groups such as emotionally disturbed versus well adjusted children. It is recommended that the KFD be used as a tool to gather information about a child's view of self in relationship to family members.

KINETIC SCHOOL DRAWING (1985):

The Kinetic Drawing System (Knoff and Prout, 1985) was comprised of the KFD as well as a new assessment, the Kinetic School Drawing. The KSD measured the child's self-concept, peer relations, and academic potential. The manual included several case examples that were helpful when interpreting drawings. Overall, the manual was easy to read and clear. Interpetation of the KSD may be difficult. Normative information was lacking. The authors did not provide guidelines for interpreting the drawings completed by special populations.

The reliability of the KSD was not established in the manual. Andrews and Janzen (1988) did create a scoring guide, reference sheet, and rating scale that demonstrated some reliability. Additional information regarding the stability of the this assessment was needed. Overall, the KSD did demonstrate some concurrent validity with achievement measures. Discriminant validity information was lacking. As opposed to Neale and Rosal's (1993) findings, this author did not agree that the KSD was a valid instrument. There was not enough information on the KSD to validate its use within the school or counseling settings; therefore, this author does not recommend the KSD.

DIAGNOSTIC DRAWING SERIES (1986):

The DDS (Cohen, 1985) measured behavioral and affective states of the client through structured and unstructured drawing tasks. One advantage of using the DDS was that three drawings were be obtained in one session. Interpretation of the DDS may be difficult. Other than noting the presence or absence of pictorial characteristics, the handbook and rating guide did not provide information related to diagnostic categories. Another possible limitation was the time factor. The pressure of completing a drawing in 15 minutes may cause stress and anxiety in some people.

Research on the DDS, to date, has shown that it can distinguish between clinical populations and well adjusted individuals. People with adjustment disorders, depression, dysthymia, schizophrenia, and organic syndromes had drawing styles characteristically different than well adjusted individuals. Guidelines for the interpretation of the DDS with special populations was lacking. Overall, the DDS showed promise as tool to provide information on clinical diagnoses. More important, Cohen (1985) established reliability and validity of the DDS. I recommend the DDS when determining the status of individuals in need of clinical evaluations.

HOUSE TREE PERSON TEST (1987):

This test was designed to provide information on personality characteristics and interpersonal relationships. The HTP (Buck, 1987) utilized chromatic as well as achromatic drawings. Guidelines for interpretation were clearly outlined. Buck (1987) furnished case examples that illustrated the quantitative and qualitative scoring methods. The manual was very detailed in its approach to design, administration, scoring, and interpretation. The quantitative method of the test was complex and required additional time in determining scores. Given that the administrator was tracking a myriad of issues, the use of a stopwatch to time the client may be awkward.

Reliability and validity evidence has yet to be established for the HTP. Some interrater reliability evidence was provided by a few researchers (Marzolf & Kirchner, 1972). Validity evidence was mixed. Buck (1987) recommended that the HTP be used as a screening device to measure maladjustment, appraise personality integration, and identify common personality characteristics of a specific population; yet, he did not provide evidence that the HTP was a valid device for screening in these areas. Additionally, he stated that the HTP can be used for employment and placement purposes. If the HTP was to be used to determine job classification decisions, evidence of differential prediction among job positions should be documented. Since the standardization sample was questionable, caution should be taken when using the HTP as a measure of intellectual functioning.

Buck (1987) was very thorough when outlining the administration and scoring sections of the manual. The case illustrations were helpful in providing insight on the use of the HTP. Another positive function of this assessment was that it incorporated color, a factor neglected by some art therapy tests. Validity and reliability evidence needs to be established. It is recommended that the HTP be used as a tool to gather information on client issues rather than as a measure of intellectual functioning. The following assessment, while lacking validity and reliability evidence, has more clinical usefulness as compared to the HTP.

KINETIC HOUSE–TREE–PERSON TEST (1987):

Burns (1987) added a kinetic component to the HTP when designing the KHTP. He found that moving figures yielded more information about client issues as compared to static figures. Additionally, combining the house, tree, and person all on one page provided more information than when viewed separately. The manual was easy to read and contained several case examples to assist the therapist with interpretation. Another desirable feature of the KHTP was the incorporation of Maslow's (1954) theory to create a developmental model for the assessment. Burns (1987) modified Maslow's approach to interpret the items on the KHTP.

The KHTP may be difficult to interpret when a symbol occurs that was not included in the case examples or the summary tables. Although Burns (1987) provided a table for the scoring of attachments, he did not include scoring information when presenting the case examples. Despite the limitations, KHTP generated some valuable information about the client's perception of herself, the environment, and her family. The kinetic component was a valuable addition to the HTP. The interaction of the items as well as the developmental model were a strong improvement over the HTP. Overall, the manual was clear and the test was easy to administer. Although validity and reliability evidence has yet to be established, the KHTP may be a particularly useful test when working with new clients. In one drawing, the therapist will gain knowledge of the client's view of self in relationship to the environment.

FAMILY–CENTERED CIRCLE DRAWINGS (1990):

Burns (1990) developed the FCCD to furnish information on parent-self relationships. Symbol systems were utilized to understand the nature of the drawings. It differed from the KFD in that the therapist was able to see the client's relationship with one parent at a time and focused in on one particular symbol. This assessment seemed to be more helpful in uncovering the barriers in the client's past relationship with their parents as opposed to discovering or getting in touch with their inner parents.

Reliability and validity of the FCCD was not examined. Interpretation of the FCCD was limited. It focused only on the drawing and neglected other aspects of the assessment domain. The FCCD was an interesting approach that generated information about the client's relationship with self and family; yet, the assessment lacked important data regarding administration requirements, interpretation, and a norm population. Guidelines for special populations such as learning disabled, hearing impaired, and culturally diverse individuals were not discussed. Overall, the FCCD had great potential as an art therapy assessment. With additional research information, the FCCD may be a valuable tool when viewing the client's relationship to herself and her family. The FCCD may be helpful in cases where the client has conflict with one or both parents.

SILVER DRAWING TEST (1990):

The SDT (Silver, 1990) was designed to assess cognitive abilities in three areas: sequential concepts, spatial concepts, and concept formation. The SDT was a creative attempt to measure cognitive skills in a nonverbal manner. Although comprehensive in its approach, the SDT had several weaknesses.

Reliability evidence was mixed. Inter-rater reliability evidence was suspect due to Silver's (1990) intervention. When using the the percentile ranks and T-score conversion charts, scores for ninth and eleventh graders were missing. This was confusing since Silver (1990) did not provide information on how to score individuals in these grade levels. The largest problem with the SDT was the lack of evidence to support the claim that the instrument was a discriminator for depression. Since Silver (1990) did not attempt to furnish this evidence, the SDT should not be used as an indicator of depression. More importantly, there was no evidence of randomized samples. Since the demographics of the sample, particularly one's cultural background, were not discussed, it was difficult to determine how the results of the SDT generalize to other populations.

Validity evidence was found lacking for this instrument, particularly the subtests, Drawing from Observation and Predictive Drawing. Also, Silver (1990) neglected to establish validity evidence for the Emotional Projection section of the test. Generally, there was no evidence to indicate what the test measures or how well it does so. Although the SDT may have limited usefulness when working with children who are developmentally delayed, I do not recommend this assessment as determination of cognitive functioning.

DRAW A PERSON: SCREENING PROCEDURE
FOR EMOTIONAL DISTURBANCE (1991):

The DAP:SPED (Naglieri et al., 1991) was developed to serve as an aid in the identification of children or adolescents who may be behaviorally or emotionally disordered. The manual was clear and concise. Administration and scoring guidelines were clearly outlined. Case examples were well structured and demonstrated the scoring system adequately. The test designers provided an excellent standardization sample that outlined demographic characteristics clearly and completely. Instructions for administration, scoring, and interpretation were very detailed, yet clear.

Construct validity evidence was weak. This was a general complaint about most human figure drawing tests (Motta et al., 1993). Discriminant validity evidence was moderate to strong. The DAP:SPED appeared to discriminate between normal populations and special populations. Reliability evidence appeared strong. No significant differences were found after a one week interval, indicating the stability of the instrument. Although the manual stated that the drawings could be used as measures of intellectual functioning, there was no evidence provided. Therefore, the DAP:SPEED should not be used as a measure of intelligence. I highly recommend the DAP:SPEED, especially in cases where a child or adolescent is suspected to suffer from emotional disturbance.

MAGAZINE PHOTO COLLAGE (1993):

The MPC (Landgarten, 1993) was designed to reveal a client's conflicts, defense mechanisms, and styles of functioning. This approach evaluated collage images as opposed to drawing style. Landgarten (1993) designed a four-task assessment protocol that was simple to administer and fit into the treatment process easily. Interpretation was based on the client's free associations and the therapist's observation of the manner in which the collage was completed. Landgarten (1993) presented clear guidelines for the administration of the MPC, materials needed, and case examples. Also, the MPC appeared to counter some of the problems inherent in cross-cultural counseling by taking into consideration images familiar to clients with diverse backgrounds.

The assessment used only images of people and inanimate objects. This limited the scope of the assessment in that animal and nature images were not considered. The fact that the MPC was to be completed in one session may be limiting. Another shortcoming was that the tasks were viewed separately. With an assessment of this nature, common themes among the tasks should be noted. Interpretation of the tasks may be difficult. The exact nature of how the collage measured transference and countertransference issues was unclear. The same holds true for the interpretation of the client's attitude from one particular image. Additional information was needed to on the interpretation of the collage tasks.

The MPC lacked validity and reliability evidence. Since Landgarten (1993) claimed that the MPC was a multicultural assessment, research should be completed to support this point. Overall, the MPC appeared to be an empowering approach when working with clients. It offered the client a choice in selection images and interpretation of the collage. Additionally, it reduced the possibility of cultural bias by including images consistent with a client's cultural background. The MPC may increase a client's awareness of self by yielding information about inner conflicts and relationships with others. It may be a particularly useful tool for therapists engaged in cross-cultural counseling.

BELIEF ART THERAPY ASSESSMENT (1994):

Horovitz-Darby (1994) created the BATA to provide a profile of a client's spiritual development. The BATA offered a free choice of art media. Given that some clients may be anxious about exploring spiritual issues, this was a valuable improvement over other art therapy assessments that were limited to using only pencil drawings. Also, the BATA can be used with agnostics or atheists. Horovitz-Darby (1994) furnished a list of questions and suggestions when working with these individuals. The manual was very descriptive and included several case examples that demonstrated the use of the BATA.

Since examiner qualifications were not discussed, guidelines for interpretation could have been more detailed. Individuals with little clinical experience or training in art therapy may find the BATA difficult to interpret. Horovitz-Darby (1994) described Fowler's (1981) theory of spiritual development in detail; yet, she did not address its application in several of the case examples. Additional information on the reliability and validity of the BATA was needed.

To date, the BATA is the only assessment in art therapy that explores a client's spiritual development. Since spirituality is an important facet of many people's life, this assessment is long overdue. As opposed to most art therapy assessments, the client was offered a wide variety of media. Although the BATA may not be appropriate for all clients, particularly disturbed clients or school children, it did offer an option to those individuals who were ready to explore their spiritual nature.

CONCLUSION

The assessments reviewed within this text represent only a few of the art therapy assessments available today. Given that practitioners differ in their assessment needs, it was my intention to provide them with a broad range of possible assessments. Family dynamics, multicultural issues, self-perception, spiritual, and relationship issues were just a few of the areas covered within this text. Although many of the assessments lacked reliability and validity evidence, some demonstrated clinical usefulness. The next chapter will present a method for utilizing and writing the results of art therapy assessments.

REFERENCES

Andrews, J., and Janzen, H. (1988). A global approach for the interpretation of the Kinetic School Drawing (KSD): A quick scoring sheet, reference guide, and rating scale. *Psychology in the schools, 25,* 217–237.

Buck, J.N. (1987). *The House-Tree-Person Technique: Revised Manual.* Los Angeles, CA: Western Psychological Services.

Burns, R.C. (1990). *A guide to family centered circle drawings.* New York: Brunner/Mazel.

Burns, R.C. (1987). *Kinetic-House-Tree-Person-Drawings: An interpretive manual.* New York: Brunner/Mazel.

Burns, R.C., and Kaufman, S.H. (1972). *Actions, styles, and symbols in Kinetic Family Drawings (K-F-D): An interpretive manual.* New York: Brunner/Mazel.

Cabacungan, L.F. (1985). The child's representation of his family in Kinetic Family Drawings (KFD): A cross-cultural comparison. *Psychologia, 28,* 228–236.

Cohen, B.M. (Ed.). (1985). *The Diagnostic Drawing Series Handbook.* Alexandria, VA: Barry Cohen.

Cummings, J.A. (1980). An evaluation of an objective scoring system for the KFDs. *Dissertation Abstracts, 41(6-A),* 2313.

Fowler, J.W. (1981). *Stages of Faith: The Psychology of Human Development and the Quest for Meaning.* San Francisco, CA: Harper.

Horovitz-Darby, E.G. (1994). *Spiritual Art Therapy: An Alternate Path.* Springfield, IL: Charles C Thomas.

Knoff, H.M., and Prout, H.T. (1985). *Kinetic Drawing System for Family and School: A Handbook.* Los Angeles, CA: Western Psychological Services.

Koppitz, E.M. (1968). *Psychological Evaluation of Children's Human Figure Drawings.* New York: Grune & Stratton.

Landgarten, H.B. (1993). *Magazine Photo Collage.* New York: Brunner/Mazel.

Lingren, R.H. (1971). An attempted replication of emotional indicators in human figure drawings by shy and aggressive children. *Psychological Reports, 29,* 35–38.

Marzolf, S.S., and Kirchner, J.H. (1972). House-Tree-Person drawings and personality traits. *Journal of Personality Assessment, 36(2),* 148–165.

Maslow, A.H. (1954). *Motivation and personality.* New York: Harper and Row.

McPhee, J., and Wegner, K. (1976). Kinetic-Family-Drawing styles and emotionally disturbed childhood behavior. *Journal of Personality Assessment, 40,* 487–491.

Motta, R.W., Little, S.G., and Tobin, M.I. (1993). The use and abuse of human figure drawings. *School Psychology Quarterly, 8(3),* 162–169.

Mostkoff, D.L., and Lazarus, P.J. (1983). The Kinetic Family Drawing: The reliability of an objective scoring system. *Psychology in the Schools, 20,* 16–20.

Naglieri, J.A., McNeish, T.J., and Bardos, A.N. (1991). *Draw a Person: Screening Procedure for Emotional Disturbance.* Austin, TX: Pro-Ed.

Neale, E.L., and Rosal, M.L. (1993). What can art therapists learn from the research on projective drawing techniques for children? A review of the literature. *The Arts in Psychotherapy, 20,* 37–49.

Norford, B.C., and Barakat, L.P. (1990). The relationship of human figure drawings to aggressive behavior in preschool children. *Psychology in the Schools, 27,* 318–325.

Silver, R. (1990). *Silver Drawing Test of Cognitive Skills and Adjustment.* Sarasota, FL: Ablin Press.

Chapter 14

AN APPROACH TO USING
ART THERAPY ASSESSMENTS:

A Case Study

Since most assessments have strengths as well as weaknesses, the most logical approach to evaluating clients is to combine several assessments. This method yields more information on client issues. Additionally, common themes may be noted by the therapist that would otherwise remain illusive if only one assessment is used. The following represents one technique for evaluating clients. This format was developed by Ellen Horovitz-Darby (1994; personal communication) to help her graduate students present a clinical evaluation of clients. The case example will demonstrate how these instruments may be combined to create a profile of a client. Lee, the subject of the example, volunteered to participate and gave his permission to use the evaluation and art work.

ART THERAPY DIAGNOSTIC ASSESSMENT

NAME:	Lee
DOB:	9/8/71
CA:	23 years, two months
REFERRAL:	volunteer
TEST DATES:	9/31/94; 10/11/94; 11/20/94; 11/29/94
TESTS ADMINISTERED:	Kinetic House Tree Person Test (KHTP)
	Cognitive Art Therapy Assessment (CATA)
	Kinetic Family Drawing (KFD)
	Belief Art Therapy Assessment (BATA)
ADMINISTRANT:	Stephanie L. Brooke, MS, NCC
	Art Therapist

OBSERVATIONS, BEHAVIORAL IMPRESSIONS:

Lee, a thin, tall, white male with dark hair and blue eyes, volunteered to participate in the diagnostic assessment. Lee stated that he worked in a plastic factory. Although he was curious about art therapy, he appeared somewhat nervous. A few times, he said that he could not draw and then would laugh nervously about what he had drawn. When engaged, he concentrated well. He did not have a marked directional preference. The quality of his strokes was soft and hesitating. Lee did not ask for suggestions or help during the session. Form was more important for Lee than color. His work was full, original, and integrated. He worked best in clay.

TEST RESULTS:
Kinetic House Tree Person Test

Lee drew his house first which suggests a need to belong to society, to have a home for nurturing, and to belong to the earth. Although he drew the last apartment he lived in, Lee talked about owning his own house one day. The apartment house has two doors, both of which seem accessible. The upstairs apartment, where Lee lived, had a smaller door knob that may represent guarded accessibility. The house contained a porch with stairs leading to the upstairs apartment. Also, the house had many windows, which may represent openness and desire for environmental contact; yet, the house contained pained windows. There was a heavy horizontal shading that separates the upper apartment from that of the lower one. This may represent the anxiety associated with the man who lived downstairs (he would often play his music too loud while Lee and his roommate were trying to sleep).

Next, Lee drew his tree on the opposite side of the page. The tree was leaning slightly away from the house indicating growing independence and moving away from family attachments. The branches were reaching up and out depicting a willingness to reach out to the environment. The tree was the largest object on the page, which represents a strong life force. The foliage was circular suggesting a possible lack of direction in Lee's energy system. Additionally, the branches were fragmented, which may characterize a person who has ideas but does not complete them.

Lee seemed stuck before he drew a gray cloud over the porch of the house. He drew his person underneath the cloud which may suggest anxiety or something "hanging over his head." He laughed nervously about what he had drawn and repeated that he could not draw well. His person was small suggesting low self-esteem. The figure had short arms, which may indicate an inability to reach out or lack of ambition. Also, the arms were stiff and may represent rigidity and inhibition. Although the figure appeared to have clenched fists, Lee stressed that they were not fists. He asserted that he drew hands but does not draw well. Lee's person was wearing a shirt that had buttons and a pocket that may depict dependency needs. The figure lacked hair, which may delineate low physical vigor. The ears were omitted on this figure, possibility suggesting "tuning out" the environment. The short neck may characterize impulsivity and stubborn tendencies. Lee admitted that he can be stubborn at times. In addition, it may suggest that separation of rational, intellectual, functioning and impulsive responsive may be difficult for Lee to distinguish.

At this point, Lee yawned, put his pencils down, and looked up from his drawing. He said he was done and we began to talk about the drawing. When we started talking about the different colors he used, he asked, "Do I have to be done now?" He wanted to work on his drawing again. He added a dog and a stick in the figure's hand. He said that the dog was his pet named Dragon. They were playing fetch. Lee laughed because he would have to chase the dog around to get the stick back. Lee was very proud of Dragon because "He was mine. I picked him out. He was my dog." When this therapist asked what happened to Dragon, Lee had tears in his eyes. Although Lee usually tells people that he took Dragon to a farm, in reality, he took him to the pound. Lee was working long hours and Dragon was couped up in the small apartment all day long. Lee did not feel this was fair to the dog. Although he tried to find a home for Dragon, he was not successful. Lee feels that he failed with Dragon, that he was incapable of taking care of him. The cloud over the figure's head may be symbolic of the guilt Lee feels about Dragon's death. This may possibly relate to Lee's physical abuse in that he was not cared for and feels incapable of caring for anything or anyone else.

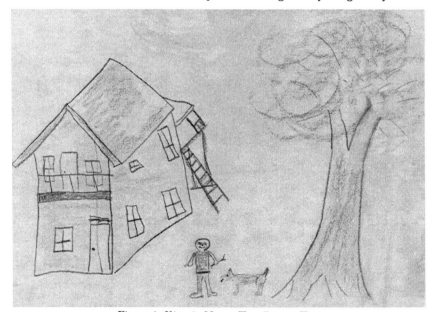

Figure 1. Kinetic House Tree Person Test.

Cognitive Art Therapy Assessment

Subtests	Scores
Drawing Response	12–14 years; pseudo-naturalistic stage Lowenfeld and Brittain
Clay Response	12–14 years; pseudo-naturalistic stage Lowenfeld and Brittain

Paint Response   12–14 years; pseudo-naturalistic stage
                        Lowenfeld and Brittain
Overall Response   12–14 years; pseudo-naturalistic stage
                        Lowenfeld and Brittain

Lee had some difficulty in getting started, saying repeatedly "I am not sure what to draw." Since he seemed concerned about his artistic abilities, this therapist provided encouragement and stressed that the focus is on how he expressed himself, not his artistic ability. Lee chose a hard leaded pencil yet drew his lines softly and hesitantly. There were some erasures on the drawing. He was able to develop basic forms and gradually became more comfortable with the process. He drew a dragon, breathing fire, on the center of the page. The dragon has sharp teeth and claws. The wings cover the body and have "thorns" on the edges. This creation was very defended. Since the neck had a lot of shading, this therapist asked, "I wonder if it is difficult for you to talk about things?" Lee said this it was true. When people push him too far, he gets angry (breathes fire). He said it takes him awhile to get to know people. Lee identified strongly with the dragon. He described it as a strong, powerful creature. He said that if he ever had a wish it would be to become a dragon. "I would do it in a heartbeat. It would be wonderful to fly, have all that freedom."

Next, Lee moved on to clay. He spent several minutes kneading and squeezing the clay. Lee was open to experimentation. He created balls, rolled them out, and made chain-line objects. First, he made a pyramid with the chains. Then, he made a volcano like structure out of the pieces. Unsatisfied with his creations, he moulded all the clay back together and then created a turtle. He started with the shell. He made holes for the legs and head and then inserted the pieces. Lee carved three claws into each leg. Next, he carved the mouth on the turtle. At this point, he stopped. He did not put eyes on the turtle, possible suggesting "tuning out the environment" or not wanting to see. His work with the clay was an attempt toward integration. Lee was highly invested in the clay. He created holes and tunnels when piecing together the turtle. He was imaginative and playful with the clay. During the session, Lee did not speak. At the end of the session, his only comment was that he liked turtles, especially their slow, easy going pace. Lee seems to adopt this pace and avoids putting undue pressure and stress on himself. Like his pencil drawing, he created another defended creature. This time, the creature had a shell to withdraw into when threatened or attacked. Whereas the dragon seems to represent Lee's fantasy, the turtle depicts his reality: Lee is a nonaggressive, sometimes passive person.

Of all the drawings to date, this was the most difficult for Lee. He never painted before and was highly apprehensive. He started out by putting small dabs of paint down on a pallet. Lee was very conservative when mixing his colors. He started drawing a pigeon in pencil and then outlined its' form with grey paint. There was separation into different areas of color (compartmentalization). Although the body was large, the bird had one small foot for support. This may suggest instability or a heavy burden to carry. The bird was streaked with color. The body was made up of the cooler colors. Yet the beak (oral aggression) andthe toes

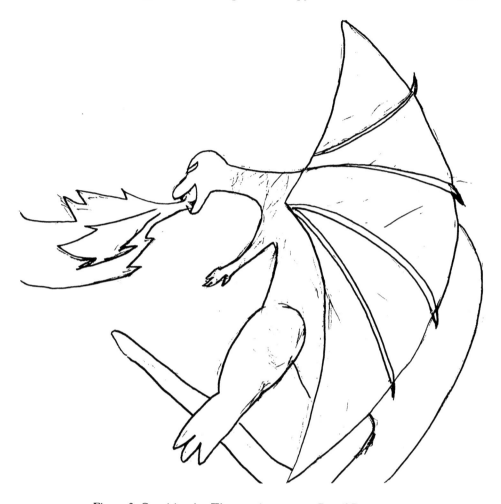

Figure 2. Cognitive Art Therapy Assessment: Pencil Response.

the toes were in red. The color red has been associated with aggressive tendencies, a theme from the dragon picture. The wing drew attention with the black and green paint. The wing seemed to be protecting the body, an image that appeared in the previous two works of art. The figure was grounded. When asked about the drawing, Lee responded somewhat defensively. He said that he just likes pigeons. "They hang together in flocks and there are always so many of them." Recently, Lee separated from his two closest friends. Each one moved to a different state. This drawing may relate to closeness he once felt with his friends.

Kinetic Family Drawing

Lee drew the shell of the house first, showing three floors. On the first floor, he drew his mother cooking. His mother had large feet possibly suggesting security needs. On the opposite side of the house, still on the first floor, Lee drew his sister

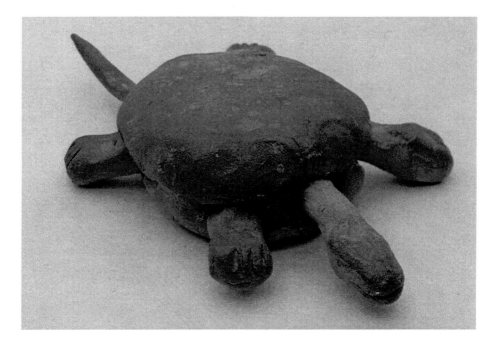

Figure 3. Cognitive Art Therapy Assessment: Clay Response.

watching television (the least important part of the drawing). Although in separate rooms, the mother and daughter were facing one another. Outside the house, Lee drew his step-father working with his tools. The step-father also had large feet suggesting security needs. Although outside, the father and mother shared the closest proximity. On the third floor above his mother, Lee drew himself sleeping. Lee was clearly separated from the family and there is no access either way. This may suggest depressive themes. For Lee, this was the most important part of the drawing. In reality, his bedroom was on the third floor of the house. Also, the roof is not closed in which would make Lee susceptible to the environment. This may reveal his vulnerability to outside influences. The closest person to Lee in the drawing was his mother. Lee stated that he was closest to his mother and fought often with his sister (who is farthest away from Lee). Lee's relationship to his step-father was ambivalent. Everyone in the family was isolated. If he could change the drawing, Lee said that he would like to draw better. Compared to other drawings, this one is impoverished.

Belief Art Therapy Assessment

Lee chose pencil to complete the BATA. When asked to depict what God means to him, Lee drew a series of images which he associates with religion. The first image was a person praying. The person's arms were chained together and he/she was crying. Lee said that a person can be trapped by their beliefs. Another image was of a cross with a nail in it. Underneath the cross were four people in

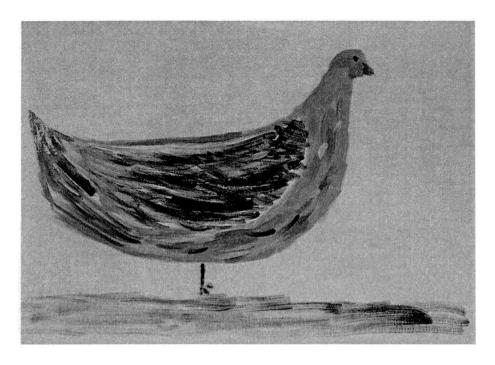

Figure 4. Cognitive Art Therapy Assessment: Paint Response.

"stressed" positions. Lee said that the church uses religion to control people and society. "Depending on how far your beliefs go, it can kill you." Another image was of a church surrounded by money. Lee felt that the only thing churches seem to care about is money. The last image was of the stone tablets containing the ten commandments. Again, Lee reiterated that the commandments were given to control people. "It is fucked up. They tell you to honor thy mother and father. Yet, what about those parents who abuse their children. Why should they have to love them back? It is not right."

Lee considered the first drawing to be his concept of religion. As opposed to its opposite, the second drawing, he felt, depicted his spirituality. He started with the image of the dragon, a theme for Lee. "From the dragon symbol I draw my strength and wisdom. When I was a teenager, I had a bad temper especially when it came to dealing with my sister. I learned from the dragon to respect my strength and control my anger so that I would not hurt people." The yin/yang symbol stood for balance in his spiritual life. The last image was of a road leading to the sunset. "This is the road of life, of discovery, and growth. Spirituality is like a journey."

As opposed to the middle sessions, Lee opened up as he did in his first session. He was very candid and expressive in his response to the BATA. Lee said that he enjoyed this exercise more than the others because it did not feel like a test. More

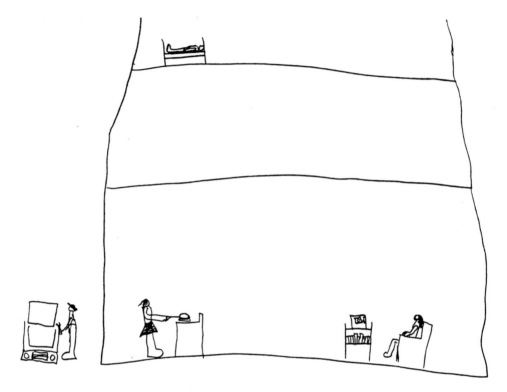

Figure 5. Kinetic Family Drawing.

important, it was related to something he felt strongly about. Please refer to Appendix II for his response to the interview questions.

SUMMARY:

Lee's work appears to be in the Pseudo-Naturalistic Stage of artistic development (12–14 years) according to Lowenfeld and Brittain (1987). Although Lee worked well with the materials, he was anxious about his creations. He was particularly resistant to working with paint. He spent about one-half hour on each exercise.

The predominant theme was that of protecting self. Lee was not confident in his artistic abilities and may suffer from low self-esteem. Given that he was unable to protect himself from physical abuse as a child, he was drawn to creatures which have natural defenses, such as turtles and dragons. Lee identified strongly with dragons and even named his favorite pet, Dragon. He collects dragons and considers them his protectors. Dragons, a source of strength and wisdom, relate directly to his spirituality as shown in the BATA. The theme of protecting self was evident in Lee's KHTP: He showed guarded accessibility in the drawing of his house. Additionally, his person stands on one foot as does the pigeon in the CATA. Another theme that relates Lee's CATA to his KHTP is extroversion.

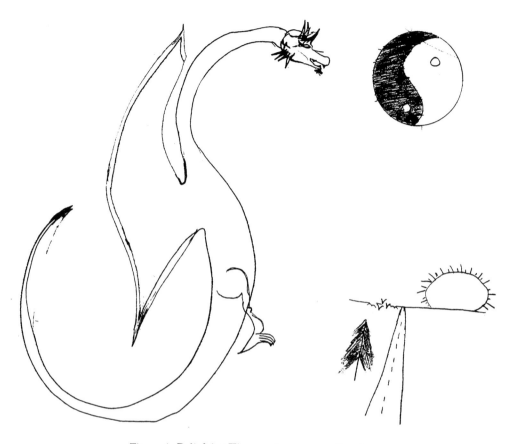

Figure 6. Belief Art Therapy Assessment: Part 1.

Lee's tree may indicate a desire to reach out to the environment as does his pigeon, a bird that he feels is sociable. In his KFD, Lee shows himself open to the environment with the open roof. This may also reveal vulnerability to outside influences.

Another theme was leaning away from the family. In his KHTP, Lee drew his tree leaning away from the house, suggesting growing independence. In his KFD, Lee drew himself two floors away from his family. There was no means of access from the family to Lee. He was the only member in the house who was sleeping which he said he used as an escape. In the last session, sleep was a prominent issue which evidenced itself in the KFD.

Lee was able to successfully conceptualize his ideas and was highly invested in the art process. He did display some initial anxiety and reluctance to using paint. This did not seem surprising since paint relates to the expression of affect, something Lee admitted to having difficulty. Overall, he demonstrated reflection and attended well.

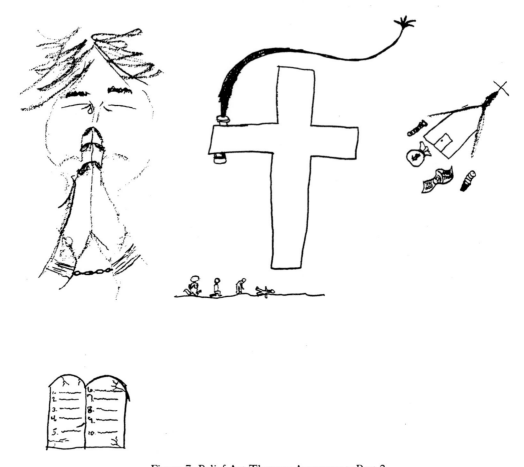

Figure 7. Belief Art Therapy Assessment: Part 2.

RECOMMENDATIONS:

Lee was very anxious about the art process initially but when engaged, he was highly invested in his work. Form was more important than color. Overall, Lee worked in the pseudo-naturalistic stage of development (12–14 years) according to Lowenfeld and Brittain (1987). This therapist highly recommends that Lee continues with individual art therapy. It is felt that the art materials and support of the therapist might provide an avenue for expressing his feelings. Working in clay may help him channel his aggressive energy. Also, art therapy may help him gain confidence in himself and improve his self-image.

Stephanie L. Brooke

Stephanie L. Brooke, MS, NCC
        Art Therapist

REFERENCES

Horovitz-Darby, E. (1994). Personal Communication.
Lowenfeld, V., and Brittain, W.L. (1987). *Creative and Mental Growth.* 8th ed. New York: Macmillan.

APPENDIX I

BELIEF ART THERAPY ASSESSMENT INTERVIEW

Stephanie (S): What is your religious affiliation?
Lee (L): Protestant, although we did not have much to do with church.

S: Have there ever been any changes in your religious affiliation?
L: Yes.

S: When did these changes take place and what were the circumstances that caused this change?
L: The fact of actually seeing what it is and what it stands for caused me to change. Protestant philosophy is that you can do what you want, and go to heaven as long as you don't do anything major like kill someone. It is not required that you go to church. Seeing the manipulation and the control factor, misuse of power, caused me to pull back more from the belief of religion.

S: What is the level of your present involvement with your church, temple, or faith community?
L: None.

S: Yet you say you are spiritual. How would you characterize your spiritual life?
L: The same way that the American Indians are spiritual. The belief in their own inner strength; the possibility of several gods instead of one; god of the sky of the earth and the spirit of the animals, things like that.

S: What is your relationship with your pastor or minister?
L: None.

S: Do you have any religious/cultural practices that you find particularly meaningful?
L: No. Just the things that are of what I am or who I am. Like, going for walks in the woods and stuff. Obviously, if it makes you feel good and makes you happy it is uplifting for your spirit. Like eating ice cream, it makes you happy and therefore it is spiritual. If you violate or hurt someone else, it is not right. The catholic church finds it ok to molest little boys and that is ok. The church just reassigns them and slaps them on the wrist. Why isn't punishment included with them.

S: What kind of relationship do you have with God?
L: None. I have a strong relationship with my spirituality. I feel I understand myself very well.

S: What gives you special strength and meaning in your life?

141

L: Dragons. Just they help give me the knowledge to make myself stronger and better. The characteristics of dragons, the properties of magic, physical strength, the wisdom, you figure that it is immortal, you will learn an awful lot if you live forever.

S: Is God involved in your problems? Do you blame God for your problems?

L: Most of them he is not. Most problems I have I create for myself. If he is involved in them he does a good job of turning my life into shit. He does things in my life to make . . . God helps those who help themselves, well I don't see anything he has given me. People say I'm strong, healthy, with people who care about you but I don't feel that those are gifts from God they are things I gave myself. I take care of myself and I have done things for my family so they love me. I work very hard to achieve my job level, which is not a lot in my opinion, it is not gifts, it is hard work. Anybody can achieve things if they work hard to achieve a goal. When an armored car crashes into my house and spills money all over the place, I will consider that a gift from God.

S: Have you ever had a feeling of forgiveness from God?

L: No. From my grandfather. There is a big difference from my grandfather and God unless someone did not tell me something when I was growing up. It was spiritual because it happened after he was passed away.

S: How was it spiritual?

L: He found a way to send a message when I felt depressed and felt that I screwed up. He tried to tell me that everything was going to be OK.

S: What form did the message take.

L: I felt a hand laid upon my shoulder and there was nothing there. I just felt his presence and I just knew who, why and what.

AUTHOR INDEX

143

SUBJECT INDEX

A

Abuse,
    Physical, 33, 63
    Sexual, 20, 33–35
Achievement, 15, 22, 30, 41–43, 87
Action, 24, 25, 31, 32, 41
Aggression, 17, 18
Alzheimers, 52
Approachers, 68, 69, 71
Art therapy assessment
    Defined, v, vi, vii, 4–6
    Validity, 5
    Reliability, 5
Attachments, 69–72
Avoiders, 68, 69, 71

B

Behavior disorders, 28, 29, 32, 44, 93, 94, 97,
    98, 106
Belief Art Therapy Assessment (BATA), 112–
    118, 126, 127, 129, 134–138, 141, 142
    Validity, 116
    Reliability, 116
    Interpretation, 115

C

Children's Diagnostic Drawing Series (CDDS),
    52, 53
Cognitive Art Therapy Assessment (CATA),
    117, 129, 131–135
Color assessments, 47–66, 112–118
Compartmentalization, 25, 28, 32, 35, 132
Cookbook approach, 6, 27, 80, 109
Creativity, 32, 33
Cultural Differences, 20, 30, 31, 35, 43, 62, 63,
    97, 98, 103–111

D

Depression, vi, 50, 51, 54, 83, 84, 86, 87,
    89–92, 106
Diagnostic Drawing Series (DDS), 47–55, 121,
    122
    Validity, 50
    Reliability, 50
    Interpretation, 49
Diagnostic Systems Manual (DSM), 47, 48, 52
Draw A Man Test, 87
Draw A Person Test (DAP), 67, 93–102, 125
    Validity, 96–98
    Reliability, 98
    Interpretation, 96
Draw A Story Test (DAS), 89, 90
Drawing analysis form, 49, 52

E

Eating disorders, 52, 78, 104, 115
Edging, 25, 28, 32
Emotional disturbance, 28, 29, 32, 35, 43, 60,
    61, 64, 93, 94, 97–99, 101, 106, 113, 115
Emotional indicators, 13–17, 20, 96
Encapsulation, 25, 30, 32, 34, 35

F

Family Centered Circle Drawings (FCCD),
    75–82, 123, 124
    Validity, 79
    Reliability, 79
    Interpretation, 78–79
Figure size, 19, 25, 31, 32, 40, 42, 43, 45, 78,
    96
Free pictures, 48, 50, 51, 105